P9-CPV-248

THE BEAUTY TRAP

the Beauty trap

EXPLORING WOMAN'S GREATEST OBSESSION

NANCY C. BAKER

FRANKLIN WATTS 1984 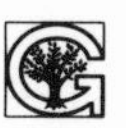 NEW YORK / TORONTO

Library of Congress Cataloging in Publication Data

Baker, Nancy C.
The beauty trap.

Bibliography: p.
Includes index.
1. Beauty, Personal. I. Title.
RA778.B2112 1984 302.5 84-7554
ISBN 0-531-09848-6

6 5 4 3 2 1

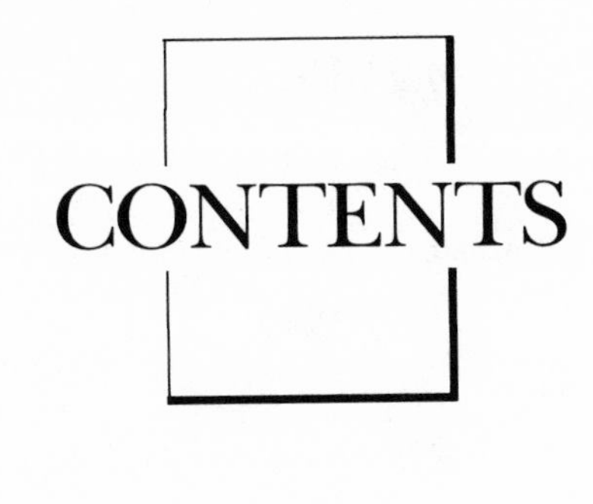

CONTENTS

Table of Contents

The contributions of experts from a variety of fields, including psychology, sociology, medicine, the mass media, history, theater, fashion and beauty, were invaluable to me in researching and writing *The Beauty Trap.* Among those who generously shared their time and thoughts with me are Laura Sinderbrand, Laura Schlessinger, Madeline E. Heilman, J. Michael Doyle, Patricia Keith-Spiegel, Lois Lee, Walter Maksimczyk, Gretchen Cryer, Norma Hertzog, Albert Stunkard, Anita B. Siegman, Jeannette Walton, John Casablancas, Kaylan Pickford and Tracy Hill.

I would also like to thank Martha Humphreys, Carol Kerner, Antoinette Lee Marangella and Judith Moll, all of whom spent numerous hours discussing the concept of the beauty trap with me. Their thoughtful comments and perceptions helped me crystalize my thoughts on the subject.

The suggestions of my editor, Ellen Joseph, helped shape the manuscript in a variety of positive ways, as did those of my literary agent, Jean Naggar, who has been faithful and tireless in her support of this project.

Countless others have my gratitude as well, although their names do not appear in this book. They are the dozens of women who candidly told me intimate details of their lives and the ways in which beauty and physical self-image have affected them. Many of their experiences are included in the book; all of these women helped me understand the personal and cultural pressures to be beautiful that we all feel.

Finally, I am indebted as always to Jerry Jacobs, who contributed both a man's and a journalist's perspective about the beauty trap from the moment the book was conceived, and whose support and encouragement made my writing it possible.

Books by Nancy C. Baker:

The Beauty Trap:
Exploring Women's Greatest Obsession

Cashing In On Cooking

New Lives for Former Wives:
Displaced Homemakers

Act II:
The Mid-Career Job Change
and How to Make It

Babyselling:
The Scandal of Black Market Adoption

To all the women everywhere
who are struggling to free themselves
from the clutches of the beauty trap.

THE BEAUTY TRAP

1

THE BEAUTY TRAP

In less than five minutes, Jane Pauley would take the seat next to mine, the television cameras would turn in our direction, and I'd be on "The Today Show." My palms were damp as I smoothed the skirt of the emerald green suit I'd carefully chosen for the occasion. I glanced surreptitiously into a mirror and was momentarily surprised to see someone else's face. NBC's makeup artist had made up that face, using far more vivid shades than I usually wore. Thank goodness. How easily I could have looked as pale as death under those glaring lights.

I surveyed myself critically, making sure that my hose had no runs and patting an errant hair into place. I gripped my book firmly and waited.

Jane Pauley walked over and introduced herself. She was even prettier in person than I'd expected. I felt plain in comparison. We took our seats and began to discuss the segment, going over the questions she would ask.

A technician pinned a tiny microphone to my lapel and hid the wires beneath my collar. Two minutes to air time. I set down my book and carefully crossed my legs at the ankles—I didn't want to show too much leg.

One minute to air time. Suddenly I realized just how ridiculous I was being. There I was, about to debut on national television with a serious and important subject to discuss, and my biggest concern was how I *looked!*

My segment of "Today" seemed to be over in a flash. I answered Pauley's questions well, managed to smile and turn my book toward the camera on cue. Luckily, I knew my subject well. I should have—I'd spent a couple of years researching and writing it. And like most women, I'd also spent a lifetime worrying about my appearance, seldom believing that I was sufficiently attractive.

At that particular point in my life I was very unsure of my looks. My thirteen-year marriage was ending, and like most divorcing women, I was worried about getting back into the dating game.

I'd recently moved from the Midwest to Los Angeles, the world capital of the movie business—and the universal capital of narcissism. Everywhere I went, it seemed, I was confronted with extremely beautiful people of both sexes. How could I compete?

To complete the turmoil of my life, I'd given up a secure job in public relations to be a free-lance journalist. Supporting myself and my young son during the financial and emotional extremes of that year had become a constant struggle.

Then the publicist for my first book—an exposé of black market adoption—phoned me. With the publication date only a few weeks away, she'd scheduled me for appearances on "Today" and "Donahue" as well as on several dozen other shows in six cities. My stomach clenched. Me? On television? I hadn't "performed" since I was in a high school production of *Anastasia.*

I called a few friends, seeking moral support. "What are you going to wear?" one friend asked. Another suggested that I'd better do something about my makeup. I seldom wore more than could be applied in thirty seconds. Still another offered to help me shop for a new wardrobe.

My first concern had been about what I would say. Would I make a fool of myself if Phil Donahue hit me with one of his famous tough questions? Would I forget all my research when the camera's red light blinked on? My friends weren't worried about that aspect: I knew my material, they reassured me. They were far more concerned about how I would *look* sitting beside Jane Pauley.

Suddenly the full realization hit me. How *would* I look? What I saw when I peered into my mirror was an ordinary, if taller than average, blonde whose skin wouldn't tan and whose hair was irredeemably straight. I did not see a double for Lauren Hutton or Cheryl Tiegs.

As I prepared for that publicity tour, I felt that my physical appearance had become supremely important, and I realized how thoroughly inadequate I thought it was. I joked about hiring Candice Bergen to stand in for me. But now I was terrified not because I feared saying something stupid but because I feared looking ugly. Women—particularly on television—are expected to be attractive, and I was afraid that I just couldn't measure up. Furthermore, I began to believe that if I *were* a Candice Bergen look-alike, my book would surely become a best seller and I a famous and successful author.

After "Today," I was kept so busy that I didn't have much time to worry about how I appeared on camera. With each day scheduled for as many as six or seven shows in a strange city, I had all I could do to get from one to the next with enough time left over to comb my hair. As I was able to handle a number of appearances without falling apart, my confidence gradually returned. And as long as I didn't actually watch myself on television, I managed not to dwell on how I looked.

When I returned home to Los Angeles, however, I asked

my friends to watch me on local shows and critique my performances. "How did I do?" I asked.

"I wouldn't wear that burnt orange suit if I were you. You'd look better in blue or green."

"But did I look intelligent? Did the show make you want to read my book?"

"Oh, sure. But do something about your hair. It hides your face when you lean forward."

So much for ignoring my appearance. My paranoia resurged.

Several of the shows had been taped, so for the first time I saw the broadcasts. Watching myself was torture. My answers to the interviewers' questions were adequate, but I worried about every one of my facial expressions and compared myself unfavorably with each female interviewer. I criticized my posture, my makeup, my clothing, my hair. I wanted to consider myself breathtakingly beautiful, yet I dwelled on my physical flaws.

Even when people complimented me I didn't feel good. I became convinced that they were merely flattering me. *I* knew I didn't look great. I looked like me . . . and that just was not good enough.

I became ensnared in the beauty trap.

Influenced by my social conditioning and my friends, but most of all by my own feelings of physical inadequacy, I let my appearance assume far too much importance in my life. I attached unrealistic expectations to beauty. And, when I looked in the mirror, I didn't like what I saw.

What I've learned in the more than five years since that time is that most women are caught in this kind of trap, some of us more tightly than others.

My friend Helen is an example. Two years ago, when she was in her early thirties, her husband walked out on her. Despite his protests, Helen convinced herself that the real reason he'd left was because she was no longer the pretty girl he'd married, because she'd gained a few pounds or hadn't taken enough care with her hair and makeup.

She became determined to repair the damage of the years. She had her hair done. She bought new clothes, perfume, jewelry, makeup. She began to diet. Once she started, however, she couldn't stop. She became obsessed with her appearance. Eventually, weighing less than eighty pounds, she began therapy for treatment of anorexia nervosa.

"I know I'm vain," she confesses. "I don't want to be that way, but I'm scared. I'm afraid to be alone and, no matter what I tell myself, I *feel* convinced that my looks are the only thing that will find me another man."

Like all anorexia victims, Helen suffers from a grossly distorted self-image. When she looks in the mirror at her emaciated frame, she sees an obese woman. Ironically, before she became so obsessed with her appearance, Helen was very attractive—a petite brunette with sparkling eyes. And she is certainly intelligent. Helen was an honors graduate of New York University and had worked for years as an investment counselor.

Although Helen's attitudes have become extreme, they're basically an exaggeration of those we all hold. Despite her intelligence, her accomplishments, her personality, and the reassurances of those who love her, she believes that her value as a woman resides in her beauty—that her only real power depends upon preserving her physical attractiveness. Because she is now painfully thin, her self-beautification efforts have actually diminished her looks.

With beauty, Helen believes that she will have everything a woman needs. Without it, no matter what else she accomplishes, she believes she will be a failure as a woman. Helen has fallen into the beauty trap.

"Beauty? I'll tell you what my beauty got me," said my childhood friend Ruth. "It got me married and out of the house at seventeen—married to a jealous drunk. That's *all* it ever got me." Ruth was the prettiest girl in high school when she married her childhood sweetheart. Now in her late thirties, she feels stuck.

"George still watches me constantly. Who am I going to run off with, I ask you? The postman? I want to leave him, but how can I? I have never earned any money of my own—George saw to that. I didn't even graduate from high school." She added, bitterly, "I don't even have my looks anymore."

Today, Ruth's main regret is that she wasn't able to prevent her daughter Kimberly from making the same mistakes. "Kim did the same stupid thing I did. Married a boy with no future to get out of the house. Eighteen years old, impressed with herself because the boys paid her so much attention. At that age, if you're pretty, it's easy to feel important. You don't realize what you're getting yourself into."

Because they were blessed with physical beauty, and because they believed it was all they would ever need, Ruth and Kimberly became caught in the beauty trap.

My friend Lucy recently had a bitter argument with her mother because Lucy refuses to lie about her age. "This is totally ridiculous. I happened to mention to Mother's bridge club that I'd just celebrated my fortieth birthday. I'm not ashamed to be forty. But Mother blew up. She didn't want her friends to know she was old enough to have a forty-year-old daughter. Who does she think she's kidding? She's *seventy-three,* for heaven's sake!"

Lucy's mother, even in her later years, is caught in the beauty trap.

Marian, a widow who's just over fifty, decided that a face-lift would help her find a second husband. So she used part of her late husband's life insurance, three thousand dollars, for the operation. "Don't I look wonderful?" she asked me after her bruises had healed. "I feel ten years younger." To me, she looked nearly the same as she had one month and three thousand dollars earlier, but I didn't tell her that. I told her she looked great.

Marian found a new husband. Ralph is sixty and he adores her. My hunch is that it wasn't Marian's new face that attracted him, it was her new self-confidence. She was lucky; thousands of women who expect cosmetic surgery to change their lives end up disappointed—and broke.

Marian, too, is caught in the beauty trap.

Satirist Ambrose Bierce once said, "To men a man is but a mind. Who cares what face he carries or what he wears? But a woman's body *is* the woman." Indeed! I'm sure no woman wants to consider herself merely a body. Yet somehow our physical appearance seems to be so much more important to us than a man's is to him. Perhaps the way to counteract Bierce's statement is to value ourselves for our minds, and for our accomplishments, as men do.

Having an improved sense of our own value, knowing that we are contributing far *more* than our beauty to society—knowing that we are, indeed, more than our bodies—should free us from the beauty trap. Yet, despite women's liberation, we clearly are not free. In the last decade we have ventured out of our homes and into the universities and workplaces in record numbers. We've made our way into business, government, education. We've earned and managed our own money, learning to be far more independent and self-sufficient. We've used our intelligence and we've accomplished a great deal.

During these same ten years, however, our purchase of cosmetics has increased by 10 percent each year, the number of plastic surgeries performed on us has more than doubled, the diet fad has grown into a $14-billion-per-year industry, and anorexia nervosa and bulimia have reached epidemic proportions. Obviously, as we have gained independence, beauty has not become less important to us; it's become *more* important. Despite the changes we've made in our lives, do we really believe, in our hearts, that Bierce was right?

As I mulled over these issues, I realized that freeing ourselves from the beauty trap is something that every woman must accomplish if she is ever to be content with herself. From our infancy, society teaches us to walk directly into the clutches of the trap. We are taught to value beauty in ourselves above all else, and we are handed unachievable standards of physical perfection against which to measure ourselves. When we fail to measure up, we begin to feel that there's something terribly wrong with us. We learn to hate ourselves. Unless we recognize what's happening and learn how to free ourselves, the only logical result of the beauty trap as we grow older—and further from that standard of physical perfection—is increasing self-loathing.

As I realized what was happening to my friends and myself, I decided that we needed to update our definition of beauty. I would explore the meaning of beauty in women's lives, and search for a way out of the entrapment. My goal was to find out how we can learn to love and accept *all* of ourselves, including what we see in our mirrors.

I began by talking with women from all parts of America, as well as from Latin America, Europe, and the Middle East. What I found was that the beauty trap has no boundaries. It's universal. There are women everywhere who are overly concerned about physical appearance and its impact on their lives. (I have changed the names and identifying characteristics of certain women whose stories are included in the book, but all other factual material is true.)

Like me, most of the women I interviewed enjoy a certain amount of primping and making themselves more attractive. They enjoy buying clothes, trying new shades of lipstick and eyeshadow, having their hair done. Throughout history, women have sought to enhance their attractiveness. Believing that we look our best increases our self-esteem and, thus, our happiness. When beauty becomes an obsession, however, when it becomes a trap from which we cannot escape, our self-esteem is diminished and, often, along with it, our physical appearance.

When we stop to consider why certain women strike us as beautiful, it's probably not because they have the cutest noses, shiniest hair, or shapeliest legs. It's more likely that their entire persona—their personality as well as (or even more than that) their physical appearance—appeals to us. As the lovely actress Claudette Colbert has said, "It matters more what's in a woman's face than what's on it."

Isn't it time that we redefined beauty for ourselves so that it includes far more than perfect physical features, artfully enhanced by makeup, hairstyling, and clothing? My own new definition, for instance, is that a truly beautiful woman makes the best of her physical assets but, more important, she also *radiates a personal quality that is attractive.* Unlike the woman with a gorgeous face and body who is obsessed with herself, my ideally beautiful woman exudes concern for others, as well as intelligence, enthusiasm, humor, and self-confidence. These are qualities we can all cultivate in ourselves, and they're qualities that will last us a lifetime.

In exploring the views of the women who shared their lives with me—some of them world-famous beauties—as well as the views of experts in history, psychology, sociology, human sexuality, business, nutrition, and anthropology, I came to the conclusion that beauty is intimately connected to the broader issues of femininity, power, and self-worth. Its implications go far beyond our ability to attract the male of our species. Beauty affects all aspects of ourselves. Because it is such an integral part of the feminine experience, and because we've been told that we all can achieve it with enough effort and enough artifice, it's much too easy for beauty to become an obsession. It's much too easy for us to believe that we are, in fact, nothing more than our bodies. By trying too hard to be beautiful, by becoming compulsive about the physical beauty we believe will bring us happiness, we actually sabotage ourselves.

We are constantly being offered a truly overwhelming number of services and products purporting to teach us *how* to become more beautiful. It's a costly lesson—we spend some $2.5 billion each year on skin care products alone. Some beauty services and products are reasonably useful, while others are simply unethical scams that profit from our unrealistic dreams and desires.

What has never been offered to us, however, is an understanding of what beauty really means to us, what we expect of it, and why our expectations often are unrealistic and self-defeating. What we really need is the ability to put beauty into its proper perspective.

This book results in part from my personal search for that perspective, from my quest for self-appreciation in all areas of my life, including physical appearance. As I spoke with people, researched the subject, and analyzed the data I collected, I realized that women must strive toward a new goal if we are ever to achieve personal fulfillment. The obstacles that historically kept this goal out of reach are disintegrating. Most of the barriers that remain today are within ourselves. When we learn to recognize them, we can destroy them.

For the first time in history, we can learn to feel—and be—beautiful. Just the way we are.

2

PERSPECTIVE ON PRETTINESS

Never completely satisfied with what nature bestows, we women probably have been trying to make ourselves more beautiful since shortly after time began. Over the centuries, we've willingly painted, powdered, scented, dyed, corseted, slimmed, fattened, paled, tanned, and shaved ourselves—all in the pursuit of an ever-changing standard of beauty.

Altering our physical appearance to conform to whatever is the current ideal of beauty certainly has cost us a great deal of time and money. Sometimes it has even cost us our health and happiness. Yet there has seldom been an era when women have not been concerned with beautifying themselves.

Probably the basic psychological reason why we've gone to all this trouble for all this time was best defined by Charles Darwin some hundred years ago. Darwin wrote that the purpose of beauty is to attract a mate and, thus, assure the perpetuation of the species. In the animal world, as Darwin and others have observed, there are certain characteristics in each species that attract the male to the female. In some species it might be nothing more than the odor of the female in heat. And in higher species, perhaps, as Darwin pointed out, it's whatever the animal considers to be beautiful.

In human beings, the sexually attracted male's first impressions certainly do appear to be based largely upon physical appearance. If we're a step or two above our animal brethren, of course, we'd like to think that the male's *second* impression of the female he covets might include some of her more lasting attributes—personality or intelligence or kindness. Still, that mythical and mystical quality—physical attraction, sex appeal, animal passion, whatever you want to call it—can't be ignored. And physical beauty seems to have a lot to do with it.

The female, like the male, has her own instinctual urge to perpetuate the species, but traditionally she also has had another just-as-vital reason for wanting to attract a mate—her basic survival. She has needed his protection from the elements and from other predatory males, and she has needed his economic support. Without him, she and her offspring might well have perished. So the message for women became clear early in time: attract a mate or perish.

But if her society tells her that *being beautiful is the only way she can attract a mate,* what is woman's future if she isn't pretty? Surely physical beauty, in its purest sense, is something we're either born with or not. After all, our physical features are largely determined by a combination of heredity and luck.

Fate is the determining factor.

Obviously women throughout history resented being the pawns of fate. Since society didn't usually allow them to find other ways to survive, either through accumulating power of their own or by using qualities other than their beauty to attract a mate, they clung to the next best hope—that they could achieve physical beauty through artifice. And their efforts to improve upon nature's gifts gave them a feeling that they were controlling their own fate.

In recent years, of course, women have had far more opportunity to achieve power than ever before, but many of us still feel we would perish tomorrow without male support and protection. Despite evidence to the contrary, we still—at the core of our being—believe that beauty is the primary, if not the only, quality that will attract a mate. So, despite many positive changes for women, many of us remain caught in the beauty trap.

There are other reasons, too, for the pursuit of beauty. Beauty is very much a status symbol, for instance. The most beautiful and fashionable women are envied by the less fortunate. And who among us wouldn't like to be envied? The wealthy, incidentally, have always been the most avid pursuers of beauty. They have more money and leisure time to do it. It's hard to keep your fingernails perfectly polished if you're working on an assembly line.

Also, beauty often assures economic benefits far beyond mere survival. Folklore has it that the more beautiful the woman, the wealthier the man she can attract. Some women earn their incomes at least in part because of their beauty, working as entertainers and models, or, of course, as prostitutes. Women have also learned to earn money by selling beauty products to other women.

There are dozens of personal reasons for wanting to be pretty as well: perhaps competition with a mother or sister, wanting public attention, or simply a belief that getting through life just isn't as much hard work for beautiful people as it is for the rest of us.

So today, as always, women have a lot invested in the belief that we can, indeed, become beautiful if we just try hard enough, that we can change what nature bestowed, that we can stop the clock. We know that it's not going to be easy. But surely, we tell ourselves, it can be done if we just find the right beauty formula. Then we'll live happily ever after.

Eve may well have been the first woman to worry about her appearance. Perhaps she stained her lips red with the juice of berries or tied up her hair with vines and flowers. Or maybe Eve was the first (and probably the last) woman to feel confident in her ability to keep her man *sans* artifice. After all, she certainly had no competition.

We'll never know exactly when women began to adorn themselves. The first recorded archaeological evidence dates back to Neanderthal women, who painted themselves with ocher and wore jewelry made of shells to enhance their appearance.

Extensive records show that the use of beauty aids in ancient Rome rivals that of contemporary women. Wealthy Roman women spent hours being primped and painted by their slaves. Although their clothing was loose and they did not corset their bodies, they used vast quantities of scents and cosmetics. Perfumes, for example, were applied to their hair and all over their bodies. Some women even used a different perfume for each portion of their bodies.

Enhancing and preserving the complexion were common concerns during Roman times, too, just as they are today. It was not unusual for a typical Roman beauty to cover her face with a thick poultice meant to keep her skin from wrinkling and to wear the concoction constantly, except when she left the house. Evidently once she was married, the Roman woman didn't feel that she needed to waste her beauty on her mate alone—outsiders had to be present before she would reveal her face.

The Romans also used depilatories, hair dyes, eye makeup, rouge, acne remedies, and tooth whiteners. The ingredients in some of these products were questionable at best. One recipe for dying the hair black, for instance, called for placing wine, vinegar, and a selection of leeches in an earthenware jug and leaving the whole mess to rot for sixty days. And we thought today's shampoo-in hair color smelled bad!

But even with such odoriferous concoctions, some of which occasionally dissolved her hair while coloring it, the Roman beauty had it easy compared with some of the women who lived in later centuries. The Roman woman, after all, wore loose-fitting clothing that left her body pretty much to nature. So if she wanted to exercise or eat or recline, she could do so without discomfort.

Somewhere along the line, however, someone came up with the notion that, just like the female's face and hair, her body, too, could be redesigned into a new notion of beauty. All it took was anything from mild discomfort to constant torture.

Perhaps the Chinese developed this concept first and best when they discovered that, by binding the feet of young girls, they could create a foot deformity resulting in a sort of natural "high heel." As the girl's foot grew, her toes became permanently twisted under the arch. The pain females must have endured in the name of beauty during the thousand years that foot-binding was customary in China can hardly be imagined. Yet some must have felt that the price was not too high. For the more petite her foot—the more tightly bound it was—the more beautiful the Chinese woman was considered to be. And, as we all know, beauty has its own rewards for women. In this case, it had an obvious reward for men, too: women with bound feet became virtual prisoners in the home, barely able to walk, much less run away from their men.

The Western world did not discover that the shape of the female body could be changed drastically until the Middle Ages, according to Laura Sinderbrand, director of the Edward C. Blum Design Laboratory of the Fashion Institute of Technology in New York City. At that time, Sinderbrand says, "Women wore dresses with bodices lacing in the front and cut close to the body for shaping that supported and lifted the breasts."

It wasn't long until the idea of lacing women into a much-smaller-than-normal waistline began to produce alterations in the feminine shape that were almost as bizarre as Chinese foot-binding. In the late sixteenth century, for example, women bound themselves into corset-bodices of stiffened canvas and whalebone. These devices featured a rigid busk (like a small board) made of wood, whalebone, or metal running down the front, which flattened the breasts and abdomen, kept the trunk straight, and drastically slimmed the entire upper body. Breathing was difficult for the wearer and bending at the waist virtually impossible. Over her corset, the fashionable woman of the day wore a contraption called a farthingale, a device that held her skirts out from her body, sometimes as much as six feet. The farthingale was made of bent wood or ivory pieces secured together with tapes, and it made the woman's silhouette look as though she were wearing a bushel basket on each hip underneath her skirts. The farthingale was worn in conjunction with many petticoats.

It must have taken women of the late sixteenth century hours to dress and, once fully costumed, such mundane activities as sitting or using the bathroom were certainly restricted, if not impossible. But wait, things got even worse. The queen of France, Catherine de Medici (1519–89), is said to have prescribed the ideal waist measurement of the day to be *thirteen inches!* It's true, of course, that women of four centuries ago were shorter and lighter than we are today, but not that much shorter and lighter. In order to achieve this epitome in waist-binding, the iron corset, a torture device that Queen Catherine is credited with introducing, was invented. It featured an entire bodice made of iron bands, like a suit of armor, hinged on one side and fastened with a clasp on the other.

Laura Sinderbrand points out that we can see parallels throughout history between fluctuations in the economic and social freedoms that women enjoyed and changes in their modes of dress. "In the decades when women were most repressed by the culture, they were most expressive in their physical appearance." On the other hand, "in those decades when women believed themselves to be emancipated socially, the shapes of their hair and dress closely followed the shape of the body and head." During Elizabethan times, women were extremely repressed socially, which was reflected in their wearing of restrictive corseting and broad skirts and their exaggerated concern with their hairdos and toiletries.

Unfortunately, the eras when women had any real power in their own right were few during the following three centuries. And, as the theory supports, this time period was the heyday of lacing and corseting women into unnatural and uncomfortable shapes. Women also often affected hairdos that took hours and hours of their servants' time to arrange. Between the vast skirts they wore and the elaborate hairstyles, often made larger with false hairpieces and wigs, the women typically dwarfed the men who accompanied them to social engagements. "As women took up less political and social space, they took up more physical space," explains Sinderbrand. "It's a rather singular way of being seen."

Although the shapes that were considered fashionable varied during subsequent years, women continued wearing space-grabbing costumes, thus assuring themselves that no one could crowd them physically the way they were being crowded politically and socially.

In the seventeenth century, the farthingale was abandoned in favor of the crinoline, which gave the skirt a more circular shape. And breasts came back in fashion. The waist was still laced to ridiculous extremes, but above the corset breasts were uplifted and enhanced.

In the eighteenth century, tremendous technological advances made fabrics easier to manufacture and dye and an age of elegance was born. But women were still restricted politically and socially and their clothing reflected their second-class status.

Toward the end of that century, elite American women like Martha Washington dressed in a very opulent style. Both men and women about the time of George Washington's inauguration wore elaborate clothing, wigs, and makeup, but the women's preparations took far longer than the men's. Popular at the time was a ghostly pallor—perhaps as a sign that a woman never labored outdoors, like a slave, where her skin might darken. That pale complexion was helped along with a notorious makeup, ceruse, which was actually a white lead-based paint known to be toxic. Despite tales of women who not only ruined their complexions but suffered slow deaths as a result of using ceruse, the practice remained popular.

Hairdos were often made unnaturally white, too. Men were likely to have their hair curled and powdered daily in a special home "powdering room" constructed just for that purpose. Women's hairdos were more elaborate, however, so they had to last far longer than a day. Their coiffures took hours to create and had to stay arranged for several months. Believe it or not, women neither brushed nor washed their hair in between these rather infrequent dates with the plantation "hairdresser."

Not much later, during the early nineteenth century, however, we can see a short-lived example of women in at least one country enjoying a relatively great amount of social freedom . . . and their clothing reflected their change in status. Laura Sinderbrand notes that the French, following the Revolution, extended their notions of liberty, equality, and fraternity to include women, at least to a greater degree than ever before. "As a result, women came out of those heavily boned corsets." Their clothing sought to emulate the classical period of the Greeks.

Portraits of the empress Josephine illustrate the favored style of the day—*Empire* gowns that were close-fitting over the bust but fell loosely just below. "They wore thin fabrics, flat-heeled shoes and a very light, unboned corset," Sinderbrand says.

Alas, this period of relative freedom for women was not to last. By the mid-nineteenth century, women were feeling the brunt of the repression of the Victorian era. And their clothing reflected their lowered status. Their skirts were once again voluminous: A well-dressed woman wore three or four petticoats during the daytime and as many as seven or eight for an important social occasion. The sheer weight and warmth of their underwear was thoroughly oppressive. Above the petticoats, their bodies were back in corsets with stays. As the century progressed, the corseting got more rigid, more tightly laced.

The following letter from a young girl who knew the tortures of tight lacing illustrates the practice rather graphically. It appeared in the *Englishwoman's Domestic Magazine* in May, 1867: "I was placed at the age of fifteen at a fashionable school in London, and there it was the custom for the waists of the pupils to be reduced one inch per month until they were what the lady principal considered small enough. When I left school at seventeen, my waist measured only thirteen inches, it having been formerly twenty-three inches in circumference. Every morning one of the maids used to come to assist us to dress, and a governess superintended to see that our corsets were drawn as tight as possible. After the first few minutes every morning I felt no pain, and the only ill effects apparently were occasional headaches and loss of appetite. I should be glad if you will inform me if it is possible for girls to have a waist of fashionable size and yet preserve their health. Very few of my fellow-pupils appeared to suffer, except the pain caused by the extreme tightness of the stays. In one case where the girl was stout and largely built, two strong maids were obliged to use their utmost force to make her waist the size ordered by the lady principal—viz., seventeen inches—and though she fainted twice while the stays were being made to meet, she wore them without seeming injury to her health, and before she left school she had a waist measuring fourteen inches, yet she never suffered a day's illness."[1]

Professionals soon began to disagree with this young woman's assumption that the custom of tight corseting was not injurious to health. Doctors protested that the corsets caused organ displacement. The clergy spoke from their pulpits against the contraptions, noting that, when pregnant women laced themselves tightly in order to look socially respectable, abortions were frequently the result.

Still, few people listened to the dissidents, least of all the women. Just as females less than a century earlier were willing to risk death from lead poisoning to paint their faces white, most were now willing to risk a variety of health problems for smaller waists.

They frequently endured "the vapors," or episodes of swooning, too. Once considered hard evidence of feminine fragility, the vapors were undoubtedly nothing more than the result of wearing such overly warm clothing and being laced so tightly that taking a deep breath became impossible. Whenever a woman fainted, the sensible advice was, "Loosen her stays!"

Yet many of these women not only ignored their own suffering, they perpetuated these customs by inflicting them upon their daughters. At a young age, girls like the English schoolgirl who wrote to *Englishwoman's Domestic Magazine* were laced into wasp-waist corsets in hopes that the garments would mold their rib cages as they grew, resulting in a "natural" hourglass shape.

In addition, during the latter part of the nineteenth century, a rather full bust and hipline were popular. Actress Lillie Langtry's 38-18-38 measurements were considered the ideal of her day. Many women embarked on what seems to be cross purposes: They went on crash diets to *gain* weight while simultaneously strapping themselves into smaller and smaller waistlines. A few excessively vain women were even reported to have undergone surgical removal of their lower ribs so that their waistlines could be laced even tighter.

Interestingly, most women didn't protest having to wear these mutilating fashions. "Strangely enough," Sinderbrand says, "it was the women who championed this fashion feature in their lives much more strenuously than is understandable. You would have thought they wouldn't have wanted the discomfort, that they would have seen it as another repression in their lives. But since the only commodity they had was their physical attractiveness, this was one part of their lives that they could control." So they perpetuated the fashion of the binding corset for themselves and their daughters despite its discomfort and unhealthy side effects.

Unlike clothing styles, makeup became less elaborate during sexually repressive Victorian times. "Good women" didn't paint their faces during that era, or at least they didn't admit painting them. But that didn't mean that faces were any less important as an aspect of beauty. Women pinched their cheeks to make them pinker and, in the mid-nineteenth century, they practiced repeating sequences of words beginning with the letter p—prunes, peas, potatoes, papa, prisms—in order to effect the small, puckered mouth that was so popular.

Some women used makeup surreptitiously. Others used "health aids" that served the same purpose as makeup. Many cosmetic companies, in an effort to survive the period, touted their products for their supposed healing or health-giving qualities. For example, a product called Carnation Lip Salve was sold in an 1853 edition of *Godey's Lady's Magazine* as a balm for chapped lips. While Carnation Lip Salve may well have soothed milady's chapped lips, it also reddened them as much as any of the rouges worn openly a half century earlier.

Although the general restrictions of women's clothing—large skirts and tightly bound waists—remained essentially the same for the next half century, there were many variations in details. The round skirt shape popular in the mid-1800s eventually gave way to a somewhat slimmer silhouette that featured a bustle on the back, exaggerating the rump.

And in the Gay Nineties breasts were very much in style and emphasized.

At the turn of the century, the Gibson Girl became the ideal, her hair caught in a loose knot on the top of her head and her body corseted into an S-shape.

But in the twentieth century, several events greatly changed women's lives and, as a result, their fashions. About the turn of the century, participation in athletics began to be respectable for women, and the idea of a more fit, slimmer body took hold. The French designer Paul Poiret advocated the liberation of the female figure from the corset in 1906 and helped to popularize a straighter, narrower silhouette. By 1913 the hobble skirt, a straight garment pinched in at the ankle, achieved prominence. Corsets were minimized, both made shorter and designed in more comfortable silk tricot.

These social and fashion changes were cemented and broadened by two important political events. The early feminist movement expanded, resulting in the granting of women's suffrage, and World War I broke out, resulting in women going to work.

Laura Sinderbrand explains that "women entered offices and factories to replace the men who had gone off to the armed forces. Women's lives and aspirations would never again be the same. Working and tight lacing were incompatible. The hourglass and S-shape [figures] and the hobble skirt were possible for women whose main social objective was decorative, but not for women on assembly lines or at typewriters and switchboards."

By the time World War I ended, women had tasted economic emancipation, the only kind that results in any real and lasting freedom. In the 1920s they adopted a freer, looser style of clothing that has often been described as "boyish." Indeed, the fashionable figure of the day was rather breastless and hipless. Skirts were raised to the knee, hair was bobbed, and makeup was back. The era of the corset was gone, but in its place were the panty girdle and the bandeau bra—both designed to reduce the curves they covered. Women began to diet and exercise to minimize their bodies.

However, the Roaring Twenties were short-lived, and the economic reverses of the Great Depression that followed meant that women were less likely to have an income of their own. Clothing once again became more restrictive. Costume historian James Laver theorizes that throughout history there is a correlation between corsets and a depressed economy, no corsets and economic affluence. In support of his theory, the more feminine shape was back "in" in the 1930s. Curves were fashionable and bodies were housed in a one-piece garment that combined both the panty girdle and the brassiere.

World War II brought us out of the Depression and again women were needed in the work force. Their clothing became looser, their hairdos and makeup less elaborate. They enjoyed economic and social freedom once more.

Still, when the war ended, Rosie the Riveter and her colleagues were sent back home, and in 1947, Christian Dior's New Look featured uplifted breasts and padded hips on either side of the reborn wasp waist. Sinderbrand recalls, "All during the 1950s, the breasts would be exaggerated with foam rubber, plastic inserts, spiral stitching and clever shaping to raise and separate. Strapless bras were popular. The prom queen was moving to the suburbs and the ads showed her waxing the kitchen floor in high-heeled pumps, a dress with a bouffant skirt and a hairdo to match."

The fifties' woman wore makeup that emphasized her lips, which were painted in varying shades of bright red and plum. Marilyn Monroe epitomized the voluptuous woman of the day with her prominent breasts and her pouty, childish mouth. She might not be the girl Mr. Wonderful would take home to Mother, but she certainly was the one he lusted after.

The pendulum had swung back again by the late sixties, a time of protests against almost everything: racial discrimination, the draft, the Vietnam War, the oppression of women. Laura Sinderbrand recalls, "Young men were symbolically burning draft cards and young women were symbolically burning bras. The headlines far outnumbered the burned bras but symbolic action does not gain its strength from numbers but from audacity."

The fashion of the time seemed to be almost antifashion. Long, straight, unstyled hair, blue jeans, T-shirts, no bras, no makeup. Yet eventually even lack of fashion becomes a uniform. Hair seemed to dominate everyone's consciousness during the protest era, men's as well as women's. The style for women was waist-length locks parted in the middle and hanging like curtains on either side of the face. Once again, not everyone was born with hair that achieved that "natural look" naturally. Numerous young women spent time removing the curl from their hair with chemical straighteners and their mothers' irons.

Legs were fashionable during this time, too, and when young women weren't wearing jeans, they likely donned a miniskirt, maybe even a micromini. These abbreviated fashions were made feasible by the invention of panty hose. A woman with good-looking legs could let them show now that she didn't have to contend with a girdle or garter belt to hold up her hose. A few fashion designers tried to sell women on the maxiskirt. But minis were too comfortable to give up, even though it was difficult for a woman wearing one to sit or bend over without revealing rather more than she intended.

For a while during the late sixties and early seventies, it seemed as though women, particularly feminists, had decided that whatever look came naturally was fashionable enough, but that trend didn't last, either. They soon learned that to hold a job—and achieving economic equality required that they do so—they had to conform to the dress, makeup, and hairstyling of which the business establishment approved. Not long after, career advisors told women that, to be taken seriously in the work force, they had to look as much like men as possible. Enter the dress-for-success look: a conservative, skirted suit worn with a simple shirt and sometimes even a tie. Career-minded women made certain that their wardrobe did not call too much attention to the fact that they were females competing in a man's world.

As the seventies progressed into the eighties, the theory was again proved that when women are more socially and politically liberated, their clothing is simpler and less conspicuous. In fact, it seemed as though the female body was suddenly disappearing. Never in history had there been so much emphasis on diet and exercise for women: in part, perhaps, for health reasons, but more often to achieve a figure that was thin almost to the point of emaciation.

As we will see, during the decades from the mid-twentieth century to the present, the desire of women, especially American women, for slenderness has become extreme. Ironically, just at the time in history when women are supposedly most liberated and most self-sufficient, more of them have become obsessed with reducing their bodies. Anorexia nervosa and bulimia are said to be epidemic.

Our approach to fashion today retains some of the individuality born in the protest era. It's easier to buy a good suit and wear it for several years than it was during the times when fashion designers annually told us to throw out last year's skirts because they were two inches too short (or too long). We seem to have more variety in the way we dress, in our hairstyles, and in our makeup.

Perhaps the look that is fashionable today has less to do with the currently popular dress or hairdos than with an overall physical image. Thin is definitely in. So is youth. Cosmetic surgery, which can help us achieve either of these modern goals, has become commonplace. We buy diet products and literature compulsively. The cosmetics and toiletries industry, purporting now to help us achieve a natural, youthful look, has never been more profitable.

Although most intelligent women are less inclined to follow the latest fashion trend like so many sheep, we still carry in our heads an idea of the way we *should* look. We may form this idea from our families, from the fashion magazines, from television commercials, from the movies, from our boyfriends and husbands—from all or none of these sources. It really doesn't matter. The point is that, despite our ability to survive without mates, we still *feel* inadequate unless we can fulfill a particular concept of beauty. The demands we place upon ourselves to conform to this concept are extremely high. Unfortunately, few of us ever feel that we measure up.

For us, liberated women of the eighties, that feeling can be almost as inhibiting and frightening as it was for women of earlier times who were bound into corsets and burdened with half a dozen petticoats. Like them, we have our own ways of using effort and artifice to improve upon what we consider our natural physical failures.

Just as an aside, the pendulum may be swinging back again. We're coming through a time when jobs have become scarcer, salaries have been less likely to rise, and we've heard a cry for women to return to their traditional, subservient roles. When the Fashion Institute of Technology closed its 1983 exhibition of two hundred years of women's undergarments, Laura Sinderbrand was amazed to hear about a "new" foundation garment becoming so popular that the department stores could not keep it in stock. Known as a corselette, it is shaped like the long-line bra of the fifties, boned to reduce the midriff and waist, and it features garters. Since the more repressive fifties, garments like these have been manufactured in black only and have been basically restricted to the wardrobes of strippers and prostitutes. But this new undergarment is being manufactured in a chaste Victorian print. "Now what does that tell you about where our society is going?" Sinderbrand asks.

Somehow, after more than a decade of the relative freedom of panty hose and lightweight bras, it doesn't sound like where it's going is forward.

3

THE MIRROR LIES

There's probably not a woman alive who hasn't, at least once, looked into her mirror and hated her reflection. A lucky few of us are generally happy with our appearance. Most of us, however, tend to find fault. Too often, when we look into that mirror, we don't see pretty hair; instead, we focus on a nose that's too large. We don't notice a pretty smile; we see thick ankles. We don't dwell on long, slender legs; we count too many freckles.

A recent survey of New York University students points up just how many of today's women are critical of their looks.[1] A full 91 percent of the female subjects were dissatisfied with their bodies, according to Ruth A. Linke, Ph.D., and her co-researchers.

Furthermore, it seems likely that if these students had been questioned about other aspects of their physical appearance, such as their hair or their face, the number who were unhappy with their looks would have been even greater. It's predictable as well that as these young women age they will become even more unhappy with the reflection in the mirror.

We're becoming more preoccupied with our looks all the time. A 1983 *Glamour* magazine survey reported that 55 percent of the women queried had become increasingly concerned with their personal appearance in the preceding year.[2] Among women in the eighteen-to-twenty-four age bracket, more than 70 percent reported an increased concern with their looks.

Women are much more likely than men are to be dissatisfied with what we see in the mirror. And that includes those aspects of physical appearance with which men are supposedly obsessed. For instance, a 1982 study by the Doyle Dane Bernbach advertising agency showed only 26 percent of men were worried about their hair becoming thinner, while a full 38 percent of women shared that concern.[3]

While we are standing in front of that mirror, doggedly cataloging each one of our physical "faults," we also usually manage to convince ourselves that they're as visible to other people as they are to us. Yet that's seldom true. The mirror lies to us. Seventy percent of those NYU coeds, for instance, were convinced that they were too fat, although only 39 percent of them actually were overweight by any objective measurement. (On the other hand, the male students surveyed by Dr. Linke and her colleagues were much better able to judge their body size accurately.)

We believe that others focus on our physical imperfections because that's what *we* do. Yet, when we observe our friends and acquaintances, we don't dwell on *their* unattractive features. Chances are we don't even notice them, particularly in people we like and admire. An acquaintance admitted that she was somewhat shocked to see a photograph of a close friend. Suddenly she realized that her friend was actually a rather homely woman, something that she'd never noticed before. In person, her friend's lively personality and quick wit made her compellingly attractive.

We also often mistakenly imagine that other women don't suffer from our insecurities. We believe that they know they are attractive, they like themselves just the way they are, they've gotten past the narcissistic worry that plagues us every time we put on makeup or step on a scale. After all, we tell ourselves, if we notice their attractiveness, so must they.

Chances are we're wrong. Even those women who have made their fame and fortune as great beauties often don't really believe they're gorgeous. They don't see themselves as others do. Lena Horne was chosen the most beautiful woman in America by *Harper's Bazaar* when she was sixty years old. Years earlier, Horne had landed her first job as an entertainer at Harlem's famed Cotton Club partially because of her unique beauty.[4] Yet she never thought of herself as beautiful, particularly in comparison with the other women who worked at the Cotton Club. "You should have seen the girls at the club," she says. "Now, *they* were beautiful! I was nothing more than average, and in later years when people insisted on calling me 'the beautiful Lena Horne,' I mistrusted and hated it."

The late Princess Grace of Monaco, surely one of the great beauties of this century, once said that she had felt so self-conscious as a young woman that "I almost crawled into the woodwork. I was so bland they kept having to introduce me again and again before people noticed me. I made no impression."[5] It's hard to imagine that anyone could have been introduced to the young Grace Kelly and not remember her beautiful face. Yet she claimed that she never *thought* of herself as particularly beautiful. She dismissed her looks by saying, "I think I'm quite nice looking, but that's about it." In fact, Princess Grace greatly resented being famous for her looks, insisting, "I'd much rather be known for my ability."

Candice Bergen, another woman who perennially makes the lists of "most beautiful women," feels that her appearance gives people a false and negative impression of her.[6] Her perfect blonde beauty has given Bergen an "ice princess" aura that she asserts is not her real self. "I hate it," she says. "I am almost incapacitated with fear in a roomful of people and have to work constantly not to cover up my fear by pulling into myself. Because of the way I look sometimes, people have always felt I was very remote. But my dream in life has been to be Italian." If she were dark and flamboyant, perhaps the real Candice Bergen would be more visible.

Dark and flamboyant looks, however, may seem just as large a burden to another woman. For instance, sultry-looking actress Nastassia Kinski, according to her friend Jodie Foster, hates her looks. "The funniest part about Nastassia," Jodie says, "is, she's supposed to be the prettiest girl in the world, but she thinks she's incredibly ugly. She considers herself grotesque. That's why she can't trust anyone who says they love her. It's like, 'God, if you love me, you must be a real jerk.' "[7] Sadly, Kinski's insecurities have tainted her self image.

Pretty and talented Sandy Duncan admits to being plagued by insecurity, too, suffering from a need to be perfect.[8] "I interpret a compliment to someone else as a putdown of me," she says. "For instance, if I'm in a group and someone says, 'Hey, look at that girl's gorgeous blonde hair,' I figure that means mine is awful."

Most of us have felt equally unsure of ourselves more than once, and the way we look is often the target upon which we pin those feelings of insecurity. Our appearance, after all, is our most visible characteristic. It is symbolic of our "real self," yet it also masks that inner self from other people. If we, like Sandy Duncan, aim for perfection, our appearance is often the first way we try to achieve it.

Beauty, as we will see, enjoys many advantages in life and females are taught its value and its power from an early age. So it's understandable that we believe that much of our personal worth lies in the way we look. Beauty can also help to hide what we feel are our personal inadequacies. If we secretly think we're not smart enough, kind enough, or interesting enough, we can convince ourselves that no one will notice as long as we are gorgeous enough. Dwelling on our facade can become very seductive.

As New York City psychoanalyst Theodore Isaac Rubin, M.D., says, "Narcissism masks low self-esteem—it's the woman who doesn't feel accepted the way she is who's compelled to spend the most time 'fixing herself up.' "[9]

It's when we try to live up to some elusive standard of beauty that we fail most miserably. Generally, we can't even define exactly what that ideal is since the fashion in beauty changes continually. In addition, no matter what the current fashion trend, all of us have our own personal standards of beauty. Dolly Parton appeals to one kind of person, Brooke Shields to another, Barbra Streisand to a third, and Sissy Spacek to a fourth.

Our tastes in feminine beauty are influenced by a variety of factors: our ethnic backgrounds, where we live, what we see in the mass media, even our personalities. For instance, psychologist Andrew Mathews, Ph.D., of Warneford Hospital in Oxford, England, found that a man's reaction to a woman's appearance depends upon his personality type. By showing a group of men photographs of women of varying body types wearing different amounts of clothing, Dr. Mathews learned that introverted men preferred thin women with their clothes on while extroverts preferred more substantial women who were scantily clad.[10]

Similarly, researchers at the University of Illinois asked college men to rate female silhouettes, then correlated their preferences with the men's personalities. They found that the men who liked large-breasted women were *Playboy* readers who were active in sports and dated often. The men who chose small-breasted women were submissive, mildly depressed, held fundamental religious beliefs, and drank little alcohol. The college men who were turned on by women with small buttocks were conscientious and uninterested in sports, while those who liked women with large buttocks were passive, obsessive, and full of guilt feelings. Among "leg men," extroverted exhibitionists liked women with thin legs while submissive, shy, self-abasing nondrinkers preferred plump legs. The University of Illinois results also reported that small women attracted persevering introverts while large women appealed to men with a strong need for achievement who were heavy drinkers.

While surveys such as these are interesting, those of us who are simply average—neither large- nor small-breasted, with legs that are neither thin nor plump—seem to be forgotten. And using the surveys' criteria, a woman who hoped to attract, say, an extroverted Baptist sportsman would be out of luck. She might be able to manage the requisite thin legs, but what could she do about her breasts: enlarge one to appeal to his sportsmanship, while keeping the other small to attract his religious fervor?

This concept is not much more ridiculous than the attempts we all make to conform to an image of beauty that has nothing to do with our real selves. Rationally, we have to recognize that our looks will not attract everyone, no matter how beautiful we are.

For many of us, the idea that we're physically unattractive may stem from childhood experiences, according to Laura Schlessinger, Ph.D., who is both a marriage and family counselor and a licensed sex therapist. Dr. Schlessinger says that women who are in fact pretty but don't see themselves that way "are still carrying some kind of real or distorted message from their parents that they're not valuable."

Alice Walker, who won a Pulitzer Prize for her book *The Color Purple,* dates a feeling of rejection by her father to the day her right eye was injured, blinding and scarring it and robbing her of her former prettiness.[11] Walker was eight years old at the time of the accident. Prior to that day, she says, she had often begged her father to take her along while he worked as "driver for the rich old white lady up the road." One of eight children in the Walker family, little Alice would flirt with her father, "Take me, Daddy. I'm the prettiest!" And he would.

"It was great fun, being cute," she says, "but then one day it ended." One of her brothers shot her in the eye with his new BB gun. "I consider that day the last time my father

. . . 'chose' me, and I suffered rage inside because of this."

The doctor who examined her injured right eye told Walker that she might lose the sight in her left eye as well, because "eyes are sympathetic." The doctor's comment terrified her. But, she recalls, it was really how she looked that bothered her most: "Where the BB pellet struck there [was] a glob of whitish scar tissue, a hideous cataract, on my eye." Walker feared that people would stare at her, "not at the 'cute' little girl, but at her scar." For the next six years she kept her head lowered, her eyes directed at the ground.

As a child, Walker hated the scar on her eye and ranted and raved at it when she stood before her mirror. She often prayed for it to disappear by morning. Yet she did not pray for sight; she prayed for beauty.

When she was fourteen, an older brother took Walker to a doctor who removed the scar tissue from her eye, leaving a "small bluish crater" where the white "glob" had been. Suddenly, Walker later wrote, she felt changed. "Almost immediately, I [became] a different person from the girl who [did] not raise her head. Or so I [thought]." With her head raised, she had plenty of friends, her classwork improved, and she left "high school as valedictorian, most popular student and *queen,* hardly believing my luck."

Still, well into adulthood, Alice Walker suffered from residual self-consciousness, believing that her blind eye disfigured her. As recently as 1982, some thirty years after her accident, she found herself not wanting to be photographed for a cover story in *Ms.* magazine. "My meanest critics will say I've sold out," she rationalized. "My family will now realize I write scandalous books." Finally she realized the true reason she did not want that photo taken: "Because, in all probability, my eye won't be straight."

There are a variety of influences that can hit us hard during childhood, sometimes causing us to form an inaccurate self-image. Perhaps someone makes a cruel remark about our looks and it sticks in our mind. A thoughtless nickname—

Freckleface, Stringbean, Carrottop—may scar us. We may feel we can never measure up to the ideal in the mass media. Or maybe we feel we can't compete with a pretty sister.

Academy Award-winning actress Jessica Lange admits that she's always disliked her nose, which she injured when she fell against a parking meter as a child. In addition, as the youngest of three sisters, she describes herself as "the ugly duckling of the family."[12] Indeed, lovely, blond Jessica comes from a family of beauties. Her oldest sister, Ann, a stunning brunette, was one of my college roommates in the sixties when we were students at the University of Minnesota. Statuesque Ann's fresh good looks had many of her friends, me included, feeling envious. Jane, the middle Lange sister, who often visited us, was also gorgeous. The truth is, Jessica, Ann, and Jane are all outstandingly beautiful women, each in her own right. There are no ugly ducklings among the Langes. Yet the luck of being born into a family that already boasted two pretty daughters obscured Jessica's concept of her own beauty.

Another attractive blonde, broadcast journalist Diane Sawyer of the "CBS Morning News," says that she has never recovered from similar sibling rivalry, despite winning the 1963 Junior Miss Pageant and later achieving spectacular career success.[13] "I really have a fundamental belief in the inadequacy of the way I look," Sawyer says today. She suspects that her feeling of inferiority "probably goes back to my sister, who was always so lean and elegant and lovely. I always saw things that bulged, like baby-fat cheeks and a pug nose. Every morning—when I come in for work—represents a triumph of hope over what I've just seen in the mirror."

If early childhood is rough on our physical self-image, adolescence stirs up even deeper feelings of self-contempt. "During adolescence, peer pressure to conform to the current mode becomes stronger than ever, and this input can lead to crippling self-criticism and distorted self-perception," according to Dr. Rubin.

Feelings of inadequacy can actually be physically painful during those years. We often go to almost any extreme to try to "fit in" and rid ourselves of those negative feelings. Jane Fonda, for instance, admits that during her teenage years, she wanted to be slender so badly that she resorted to taking amphetamines and diuretics.[14] Whenever her appetite got the best of her, she binged on food, then tried to atone for her "sins" by purging herself of the food—exhibiting behavior that today would be recognized as bulimic.

Goldie Hawn, on the other hand, says that she felt horribly skinny during her teenage years.[15] She sometimes wore two pair of socks at a time to make her ankles look thicker, as well as a padded bra to flesh out her flat chest.

Pretty singer-actress-model Michelle Phillips, who became famous as a member of the Mamas and the Papas rock group during the sixties, suffered as an adolescent because of her small breasts. "When I was growing up, breasts were everything," she recalls, "and I had no breasts. I felt terribly inferior because I was so small-bosomed. As I got older, [my] look came in—thank God, because I don't know if I could have survived it otherwise."

Phillips says that dwelling on what she felt was her physical deficiency gave her "an inferiority complex. As a matter of fact, I started stuttering again when I was seventeen. I had stuttered when I was a little girl and then I was fine—until I realized that I wasn't going to get any breasts."

Meeting John Phillips, whom she later married, helped Michelle overcome her feelings of inferiority. "I remember John telling me when I was seventeen years old that I was in the top one percent of beauties. I used to love to hear him tell me this. It wasn't until I met John that I began to believe that I was pretty. And then, when I started to model, I think I got more of a sense of myself."

Actress Debra Winger, who made an impact in the movie *An Officer and a Gentleman* as well as in *Terms of Endearment*, still smarts from a remark her father made to her when she quit college to go into acting. "My father told me: 'You can't be a movie star. Movie stars are beautiful.' I believed him. I thought, 'Well, you're right, so I guess I'll be an actress, instead of a movie star.' "[16] Often parents who make such remarks don't realize the damage they do to their daughters' self-esteem.

Yet, despite her father's warning that she'd never be a movie star, Winger has always felt more comfortable acting before a camera than before an audience. Her feeling that she lacks physical beauty may well be a primary reason for her preference. "The camera's nonjudgmental. The camera isn't going to say, 'You're ugly.' The camera's just going to tell the story. So it's my best friend."

Ironically, Debra Winger may have become a movie star in part because she didn't feel pretty enough to be comfortable on stage.

Actress Anjelica Huston, on the other hand, was made to feel ugly because the movie camera that photographed her when she was fifteen was critical. Cruel reviews of her first movie, *A Walk With Love and Death,* which was directed by her father, John Huston, left her feeling "exposed and unlovely."[17] Most of the reviews of the 1969 film "said I was wooden and not very pretty," Huston recalls. "I was at a particularly unattractive stage of adolescence, and since the role called for a very pretty girl, that made it very hard for me. I came out of the experience feeling quite bruised."

In subsequent years, Huston outgrew her adolescent awkwardness and found success as a fashion model. Yet she still "felt unhappy about my looks. When I was modeling, it was terribly hard for me to even make up in the same room as the other girls because they all looked so lovely with their small noses and perfect eyes." Overcoming her teenage sense of physical inadequacy was slow work for Huston. "It's taken me a long time to feel comfortable with the way I look."

For some of us, such early wounds never heal. We persist in seeing ourselves as awkward fifteen-year-olds long after we've outgrown the traumatic teenage years.

If any of us emerge from childhood and adolescence with fairly positive feelings about our looks, chances are that some later event in our lives will at least temporarily alter our perception. In our society, gaining weight, aging, and changes in fashion all take their toll on feminine self-esteem, even among women who appear to the rest of the world to have everything.

Model Christina Ferrare, for instance, found herself becoming extremely insecure about her looks after the birth of her daughter.[18] "I'd gained a lot of weight—I shot up to 190 pounds. And where I was always used to a lot of attention from men, now I would get pats on my head instead of remarks about my looks. I was so fat, all blown out of proportion. I wanted my youthful body back, and all the attention."

Ferrare, who is the wife of John DeLorean, lost the weight she'd gained, but her self-esteem didn't return instantly. She went back to work feeling unattractive to men. A long time passed before her previous confidence in her looks, and in herself, returned.

All of us, at some time in our lives, worry about whether or not we're attractive to men. Although there's plenty of evidence that beauty attracts men, holding them requires quite different attributes. We tend to forget that. So as we grow older and notice our looks fading, we worry increasingly about our sexual desirability.

Debbie Reynolds, although she's in fine enough physical shape to star in her own exercise videotape, shares that concern.

Now over fifty, Reynolds says she is looking for a man who's no Adonis. "Perfect, gymnastic, macho-looking men terrify me. And I'm too insecure to go out with a gorgeous younger man. I would always be thinking: 'He's looking over there at that beautiful young girl.' What I like is a man with a little stomach. I want something to hold on to when I put my arms around him."[19]

Even Renaissance woman Maya Angelou, who seems to have danced through her amazing life more on sheer energy and creative intelligence than on physical appearance, thinks she may need beauty to help fill her need for male companionship in her middle years. She recently told of becoming so lonely one night that she invited a male friend to visit her "so I could cry on his shoulder, and he could hold me in his arms. Instead, we had a drink and talked about my book tour. Then he went home, and I went to bed and just bawled."[20] She would like to find a permanent male companion to ease those feelings of loneliness, but "sometimes I think I'm too old or too fat. Or I wish I was prettier."

Many of us, when we peer into our mirrors, feel that all our problems would be solved if we could just change the way we look. If we could only be as pretty as Candice Bergen or Lena Horne or Debbie Reynolds or Diane Sawyer, we believe, our lives would be different.

Yet when these attractive women critique themselves—as all women do—they certainly spot their flaws. Sometimes they even dwell upon them, feeling inadequate and devalued.

Surely if such accomplished women and celebrated beauties get caught in the beauty trap, it's understandable that the rest of us do, too. All of us have a tendency to place far too much emphasis on our physical appearance. We often concentrate on our real or imagined defects, those flaws that others don't even notice. As a result, we rob ourselves of well-deserved happiness. Ironically, this preoccupation with ourselves ultimately makes us less attractive to other people.

However, we can change this self-destructive pattern. Our first step is recognizing that, like most women, we have a negatively distorted view of ourselves. We are far too critical of our own physical appearance. Once we realize this, we can progress toward freeing ourselves from the beauty trap.

4

THE PARADOXES OF PRETTY

On a cold January night in 1980, a pretty thirty-nine-year-old woman met a group of six young men in a bar in Holbrook, Massachusetts, and left with them. A few hours later, she lay naked and bruised in a nearby woods. The woman, described over and over again by the media and defense attorneys as "a former beauty queen," claimed that the men had raped her. The men claimed that she had agreed to have sex with all of them for two hundred dollars. After all, they implied, why would a good-looking woman leave a bar with six men unless she was prepared to have sex with them?

In a plea bargaining agreement, the men pleaded guilty to rape. In return for their guilty plea, the judge, stating that the situation was actually "a consensual sexual adventure that went off track," imposed suspended sentences and five-hundred-dollar weekly fines, to be paid in five-dollar weekly installments.

But the judge hadn't counted on the public outrage that followed his lenient sentence. A few days later he revoked the suspended sentences and ruled that the case must go to trial. In 1983 five of the men stood trial—the sixth testified against his buddies—and all five were acquitted of the rape charges. (They *were* found guilty, however, of damaging the "former beauty queen's" automobile.)

Vickie is the kind of young woman who's always noticed in a crowd. She's strikingly pretty in a fresh, midwestern way, with shiny brown hair, a creamy complexion, a trim figure, and an engaging smile. When she was fifteen, Vickie won her state's Miss Teenage America beauty pageant, and she was selected Miss Congeniality as well. She wasn't passed over when they handed out the brains, either. In high school, Vickie was a straight-A student. When it came to dates, you'd have expected her to be popular. "Nobody asked me out when I was in high school," Vickie remembers. "I never went to a prom or homecoming or anything." And when she got to college, *she* had to ask the men out.

Sherry Black Kozloff is attractive, blonde, and successful in her career as director of national market development for ABC radio. Yet her good looks were no help in getting her that job. In fact, a few months after she was promoted from ABC's FM division to the corporate staff of ABC radio, she received a phone call from the former president of the FM division.

"It was completely out of the blue. He called and said, 'I want to tell you how sorry I am that I couldn't do more for you when you worked for me. I couldn't do as much for you as I could for some of the men because I was afraid of what people would say or do—because you are so attractive.' "[1]

These three women, the rape victim, Vickie, and Sherry Black Kozloff, all have experienced the negative aspects of being beautiful. The rape victim learned that many people believe that a pretty woman is enticing to men, so she deserves what she gets—even if it's rape. Vickie, while enjoying the attention she received, found that men are often afraid to approach pretty females. And Sherry Black Kozloff learned that good looks can hurt a career because of the myth that beautiful women, no matter what their job qualifications, get ahead only by sleeping with powerful men.

It's true that beauty has its rewards; there's no doubt about that. Study after study has shown that most people simply react differently, and positively, to beautiful people.

It is the opinion of psychology professor Ellen Berscheid, Ph.D., of the University of Minnesota, that beautiful people are given preferential treatment in our society. Dr. Berscheid, who in collaboration with other psychologists has authored several studies on the subject, says, "Attractive individuals are generally believed to be more sensitive, more kind, interesting, strong, poised, modest, sociable, outgoing and exciting."[2]

But that's not the whole story. Beauty is very paradoxical. It is often described as both pure and evil, as both innocent and seductive, as evidence both of quality and of superficiality. While many people surely do ascribe desirable qualities to the physically attractive, they may also think that beautiful people, particularly women, possess negative traits: that they're unintelligent, that they're vain and self-centered, that they have undeserved power over men, that they lack ambition and drive, that they're fickle friends and lovers. Certainly any beautiful woman could name a dozen more negatives she's had to combat. Although most of us would still choose to be beautiful, we also may feel a touch of ambivalence about that prospect.

Perhaps those of us who possess more envy than beauty might think, "Serves her right!" when a good-looking woman encounters a negative reaction to her appearance. Even if we aren't feeling particularly sympathetic about the problems our better-looking sisters face, however, it's important to examine some of the mixed messages about beauty that we've all received. Beauty, after all, is relative, and these paradoxes affect all of us. Suppose a friend makes an effort to look her best for a blind date—maybe she buys a new form-fitting dress, has her hair done, is particularly careful with her makeup—and then encounters an unwanted and insistent pass. She is likely to be ambivalent and feel guilty. "What did I do to cause *that*?" she asks herself. What she did, she concludes, is make herself look attractive. Or what about listening to society's strong message that we should try to appear as appealing as we possibly can, and then finding we are treated as if we are beautiful but dumb when we do just that?

Taking a close look at some of the double-talk we've all heard about beauty should help us put the issue into better perspective. It should help us understand why we so often feel ambivalent about beauty and that no matter what pains we take with our appearance, we are doing the wrong thing.

> PARADOX: *A woman has the power to attract the men she needs and wants with her beauty. But men can be dangerous.*

When I was fifteen and needed to earn some spending money, I took a job as a carhop at a drive-in restaurant in a suburb of St. Paul, where I lived. During the school year I worked weekends, and during the summer I often worked nine hours a day, six days a week. I have vivid memories of the hard, physical work, carrying heavy trays for hours in weather that ranged from the high, humid nineties in the summertime to below zero in the wintertime.

But I have equally vivid memories of something else—the boys who came into the drive-in to get their kicks from harassing me. "Hey, Blondie, what time you gettin' off tonight?" one might shout at me. Another might yank my ponytail or my apron strings as I turned away from his car after delivering his food. A third might offer a shrill wolf whistle as I walked across the parking lot. I don't remember any of these boys by name or face. They all tended to look alike to me, the same greasy hairstyles, the same pimply faces, as they sat in their nearly identical souped-up cars waiting for a carhop to deliver their Cokes and fries.

This was the Midwest in 1960, of course, and drive-ins with carhops are extinct today. What I experienced then, as a naïve teenager, was surely only a fraction of the harassment that a cocktail waitress might encounter today. Some have told me that their male customers now often feel free to grab their breasts, slide a hand under their skirts, or blatantly proposition them.

Still, I remember feeling embarrassed by those remarks and gestures, and a little angry at being made into a public spectacle. If I'm completely honest about it, I have to admit that I was sometimes flattered, too. Not all the carhops got wolf whistles. I was also sometimes frightened. Even though the restaurant's owner drove all the carhops home after closing time, there was always the remote possibility that one of these boys might be waiting in the dark. I don't remember articulating my exact fear at the time, but it was rape.

There was another emotion I felt, too, one that seems in retrospect to be unwarranted. Yet the emotion was a reflex action. That emotion was guilt. A little of the guilt was over my feeling flattered. In addition, I felt that there must be something about the way I looked or walked or talked or tilted my head that *caused* these boys to act in a very disrespectful way. Perhaps their behavior was *my* fault, not theirs. I felt ashamed.

I didn't know what I could do about the situation, short of finding another job, but jobs for teenagers were hard to come by.

I have felt the same combination of emotions—embarrassment, anger, fear, guilt, shame—at other times in my life when men made remarks about my appearance, such as when an employer announced that I had "good legs" during a business meeting; when a radio interviewer told me, on the air, that I looked "too fresh and wholesome" to be from California; when a hand suddenly materialized in a crowded room and pinched the backside of my ski pants.

These experiences were unfortunate, for the purpose of this kind of public come-on is really power. A male who would shout, "Hey, Blondie, what time you gettin' off tonight?" across a crowded drive-in parking lot is hardly looking for a relationship with "Blondie." He is showing off for his friends, at my expense. And he is very clearly putting me in my place, letting me know that I am nothing but a sex object, someone who should fear his potential physical power over me.

So why couldn't I simply react with anger, an appropriate emotion to such an insult? I think it's because women have bought the male idea that our beauty is our power. According to this theory, if a man reacts to us with a display of *his* power, whether it's in the form of verbal abuse, an unwanted touch, or rape, it's not his fault. *We* caused his behavior.

In order to understand the dynamics of this situation, let's take a look at the man who displays the extreme dimension of hostility toward women—the rapist.

Timothy Beneke, author of *Men on Rape,* says that "clearly, to men, a woman's *appearance* is a weapon."[3] He notes some of the phrases men frequently use to describe a woman's looks, such as, "She's a *knockout*!" "That woman is *ravishing*!" "What a *bombshell*!" "She's really *stunning*!" All words of violence and power.

Beneke states that most heterosexual men at times have felt attacked by a woman's beauty. Her power, he says, is not so much physiological, although that plays a part. It has more to do with how men understand sex. "If sex is an achievement, then the presence of an attractive woman may result in one's feeling like a failure. One's self worth, or 'manhood' may become subtly (or not so subtly) at issue in her presence."

Such a man probably realizes that he couldn't win the beautiful woman in front of him. He feels that she would choose a man who is richer, smarter, more handsome, and he resents that. He feels without even trying that he doesn't measure up to her standards. And it becomes *her* fault that he feels inadequate.

If he's hostile enough, this man may want to make the woman feel as degraded as he does. His degrading her, depending upon the man and the circumstances, can take the form of any action from a demeaning sexual remark to rape.

In his book, Beneke quotes a young man, "Jay," who articulates these feelings. "A lot of times a woman knows that she's looking really good and she'll use that and flaunt it, and it makes me feel like she's laughing at me and I feel *degraded.* If I were actually desperate enough to rape somebody . . . it would be a very spiteful thing, just [so I'd be] able to say, 'I have power over you and I can do anything I want with you,' because I really feel that *they* have power over *me,* just by their presence. Just the fact that they can come up to me and just melt me and make me feel like a dummy makes me want revenge."

Many pretty women sense this "power" we're supposed to have over men, of course, and some use it in unfair ways. There are women who are teases and others who seduce men in order to manipulate them, just as there are women who are honest about their feelings. Yet, even those of us who try to deal with men honestly often feel guilty, as though we have used our "power" wrongly, when a man reacts to us physically in a hostile way.

I was listening to psychologist Toni Grant's ABC radio show a while ago when a young woman called in wanting advice about why she couldn't seem to lose twenty-five extra pounds.[4] It seems that the woman had gained this weight three years earlier, just after she'd been raped. For most of her life, until she entered college, she'd been overweight. When she moved to campus, she slimmed down and suddenly felt attractive and was popular. She had dates with a variety of men; then one of those men raped her.

"The rape was a terrible price to pay for being pretty, wasn't it?" asked Dr. Grant in articulating the rape victim's feelings.

Clearly the young woman felt that if she had not been attractive—in her case attractive was defined as thin—she would not have been raped. So, in order to insure that it could never happen again, she subconsciously decided not to be thin again. Being thin means being sexual and, therefore, vulnerable, Grant advised the caller. The young woman could not cope with that kind of vulnerability.

My guess is that this rape victim also felt at least partly responsible for her own fate. After all, losing her girlhood chubbiness when she entered college was an overt action, one that caused her to become attractive to men. A part of her believed the traditional male rationalization for rape: She attacked me with her weapon (beauty), so I attacked her with mine (my penis).

A feeling of responsibility and guilt for her own rape, however inappropriate that is, is not unusual for the victim. This feeling is often connected with how she has made herself *look.* If we believe that we can create beauty and that beauty has the power to attract men, then we must believe that there are consequences of this act. Not all of those consequences are pleasant.

I heard one such story from a psychologist who told me about a friend who had been raped and then spent the next several years making herself as unattractive as possible without even realizing why. The reason why, of course, is that, *if you are beautiful, you are vulnerable* to various kinds of degradation and humiliation, including rape.

Of course, all females, whether they're beautiful or not, young or not, slender or not (and males, too, for that matter), are vulnerable to rape. But what I'm discussing here is a basic fear that all women possess, that, if our beauty can be used to attract the right kind of man, there's no guarantee that it won't attract the wrong kind.

Psychologists agree that beautiful women generally are perceived as "more feminine" than less attractive women. As we will see, this stereotype causes many problems for pretty women, and attracting male hostility is one of them. If a man is basically hostile to women for whatever reason—perhaps he still resents the power his mother wielded over him when he was a child, perhaps he has been unlucky in love, perhaps he has to blame someone else for his own personal failures and women are an easy target, perhaps he simply has been reared to believe that males are superior to females—seeing or interacting with an attractive woman is likely to spark his hostility.

During my second summer as a carhop in that midwestern drive-in, I worked with another teenager, Angela. Angela, at sixteen, had a thirty-nine-inch bust, an attribute that the boys in the souped-up cars commented upon endlessly. She wore a sturdy bra and a conservative uniform buttoned up to her chin, but that didn't matter. Angela became known as "Miss Boobs" or "the brunette Jayne Mansfield" to the crowd in the back lot. Her cheeks would burn with shame each time an off-color remark was made. After perhaps seven or eight weeks on the job, she quit, unable to take the verbal abuse any longer.

Angela could hardly be blamed for her figure, and she did nothing to enhance it. Yet, she felt inadequate, embarrassed, ashamed, even a little guilty, whenever she was the butt of those uncouth remarks.

A few years later, Angela had breast reduction surgery. For her, as for many attractive women, the cost of beauty—dealing constantly with hostile men—simply became too high. Angela was ambivalent about her appearance, so she dealt with her ambivalence surgically.

PARADOX: *The beautiful woman is admired by many; but few can see beyond her beauty.*

The beautiful woman risks being *defined* solely by her beauty. Angela, for instance, felt defined by her figure. Men, and to a certain extent other women, considered her the stereotypical sexpot, not because of her behavior, but simply because of her ample bustline. Her intelligence, her wit, her ambition, even her faults were hidden to other people because they didn't see past her chest.

Vickie, the twenty-six-year-old beauty contest winner who never had a date in high school, has fought hard to make people look at the real woman behind her beautiful exterior. In high school, she says she didn't make the connection between her appearance and her lack of boyfriends. Besides, she was busy with extracurricular activities and was not that interested in dating. It wasn't until she reached college that she realized that the asset she'd been exploiting in beauty contests was causing her to be categorized in a negative way.

"It suddenly dawned on me that people just do not take good-looking women seriously," Vickie says. A broadcasting major in college, she had "professors who wouldn't let me climb the ladders and fix the lights in the TV studio. They always wanted me in front of the camera, not behind it."

Until she entered college, Vickie had felt good about her participation in those beauty pageants: "The way I looked at it was, if you have enough poise to get up in front of an audience with just your bathing suit on, you can fare well in any situation. So I didn't look at it as a cattle call or anything like that." In each contest she entered, she always excelled in the talent portion and "in almost every contest I was in, I was at least a runner-up."

Ironically, despite her trophies, Vickie didn't consider herself unusual. "I never thought of myself as either extremely good-looking or very plain. I just thought [the contests] were what everyone did." Vickie considered the beauty pageants as an arena in which to exhibit her talents more than her looks.

In college she lost her naïveté about other people's perceptions of beautiful women. Once she realized that her appearance interfered with her studies, Vickie made an effort to change. She stopped entering the contests and worked on developing a new image. "In college," she recalls, "I really tried to downplay my looks because I didn't want people to take me for my looks only. I went from wearing a lot of makeup and doing my hair and everything to no makeup and jeans and no bra. I became almost a militant feminist."

In order to diminish the discrimination she felt when stereotyped as an empty-headed, if decorative, female, Vickie tried to be one of the guys. As the only female in her major field of study, it wasn't easy for her to become inconspicuous, but she tried, even to the point of moving heavy studio equipment. And, "I used to tell a dirty joke every day," she says with a laugh. "I used to be a good beer chugger, too. That was a definite asset. It got to the point where I was more like one of the guys than most of *them* were. But that way they finally treated me like a person instead of like an object."

Being treated as a stereotype is a drawback in both our personal and professional lives, but it's probably easier to examine its effects in the work world. Several university researchers have studied physical attractiveness in business with generally consistent results.

As we might suspect, beauty can be an asset in finding a job. Businesses often prefer that a "front office" position be filled by a young and attractive female. Of course, in certain professions, like modeling, attractiveness is mandatory. Yet many pretty women who aspire to middle- and upper-level jobs in typically male fields find that what they've always been told is an asset is really a serious detriment.

New York University psychology professor Madeline E.

Heilman, Ph.D., has found that attractive women are more likely to be hired for low-level jobs, and less likely to be hired for managerial jobs. She and her colleagues asked forty-five male and female management students at Yale to act as personnel managers in a recent research study.[5] The students were asked to evaluate bogus job applicants, each applying for one of two jobs in a large insurance company. Dr. Heilman describes her study: "Each of the men and women in the study was given a description of either the managerial or nonmanagerial job and copies of four standard employment application forms, each ostensibly completed by a different applicant. In fact, the applications were equivalent in background and job qualifications. Attached to each application was a photograph." In each case, two of the job applicants were male and two female, two were attractive and two unattractive.

Interestingly, good looks turned out to be an asset for men seeking either job. But for women, the findings were different. The good-looking women were more likely to be hired for the nonmanagerial position, and much less likely to be hired for the managerial position. "They were rated as less qualified and less likely to be recommended for hire than were unattractive women with equivalent backgrounds," says Dr. Heilman. And, "to add insult to injury, when [the pretty women] were recommended, it was at a lower starting salary."

Suddenly the supposed "advantage" of being beautiful had become a disadvantage. The beautiful woman's trouble doesn't stop with applying for a mid-level position, either. In 1983, Dr. Heilman and her colleagues undertook a similar study, this one designed to appraise the performance of attractive and unattractive workers who were already on the job. "Again," she says, "we found that for women, attractiveness was an advantage in a clerical position, but a disadvantage in a management position." Attractive female managers in this second study (whose bogus accomplishments on the job were equal to those of their unattractive female counterparts) scored quite poorly. As opposed to the unattractive women managers, the pretty ones were rated lower in job performance; were judged less likely to be promoted; were thought to be less deserving of a raise in pay; and if they were recommended for a raise, the actual dollar amount of the raise was less.

Why are attractive women at a disadvantage in professional jobs? Dr. Heilman's research shows that attractive women are thought to be more "feminine" than less attractive women. "And femininity seems to run counter to popular conceptions of what it takes to do certain types of jobs well. The evidence [in the studies] indicates that stereotype thinking links femininity with indecisiveness, passivity, emotionality and other traits antithetical to successful performance in such roles. Thus, the more attractive a woman, the less suitable she appears for a job believed to demand masculine skills for success."

As both Heilman studies show, people don't let the facts get in the way of their pet stereotypes. Even though the attractive women were documented to be as fully qualified as the unattractive ones, the evaluaters ignored that documentation and assumed that they had to be less qualified by virtue of their beauty.

Many people are terribly uncomfortable with the idea that a woman can possess both beauty and brains. Frequently, good-looking women who are also smart have to work much harder to be recognized. In fact, many people prefer almost any explanation *other* than competence for why a pretty woman is successful. That conclusion is among the findings of a survey of attractive and successful women undertaken by Lita L. Schwartz, professor of educational psychology at Pennsylvania State University, Abington, and Florence W. Kaslow, associate professor and chief of forensic psychiatry and psychology at Hahnemann Medical College and Hospital in Philadelphia.[6]

Schwartz and Kaslow questioned fifty-nine attractive women in a variety of business and professional fields, including thirteen Ph.D.'s, three M.D.'s, one law degree, fifteen Master's degrees, and fourteen Bachelor's degrees. Most of these women enjoyed being attractive and they found it advantageous in certain situations, such as initial meetings with clients. They felt noticed. But, Schwartz and Kaslow note, "attractive women face an additional handicap, since it is part of our folklore that attractiveness and competence cannot go hand in hand. As a result, many colleagues assume that the attractive female professional has obtained her high-level position through seductiveness, manipulation, or because she has been sexually available. That she has acquired a high-ranking position through long years of education and training, hard work, resourcefulness, creativity, and tenacity is not given credence."

More than three quarters of the women who responded to Schwartz and Kaslow's study said that they had been the subject of unfounded gossip and insinuations at work. With that kind of atmosphere common in business, it's not too surprising that women like Sherry Black Kozloff, the ABC radio director of national market development, finds employers unwilling to promote them, even when their competence has been demonstrated fully. By helping, an employer sets himself up as a target for gossip, which might hurt his own career.

About half of the successful women in the Schwartz and Kaslow study also reported having experienced jealousy from their female colleagues. So, it seems, the attractive but ambitious woman may well find herself condemned from all sides.

Many a boss's wife has objected to his hiring or promoting a woman who's too appealing. A wife may feel threatened by her husband working closely with a beautiful female employee.

God help the beautiful woman who makes a mistake, too,

because it doesn't look as though anyone else will. As Los Angeles career counselor Adele Scheele, Ph.D., puts it, "The extra-attractive woman who faces trouble gets little sympathy from others. People will not support her because they think she already has more than her share of advantages."

The point of all this, of course, is that the beautiful woman is likely to be treated as a symbol rather than as a real person. And, whenever anyone is considered a stereotype instead of an individual, she could have serious problems. We've seen how damaging this is to a woman's professional life. It can hurt her personal life, too. Often, as Vickie found out, men are intimidated by beautiful women and dare not approach them. At least the woman, if she has Vickie's self-assuredness, can turn the tables and approach the men. But there also are many men who are attracted *only* by a woman's looks, never noticing what other qualities she has to offer. Sometimes, when it comes to relationships with the opposite sex, a beautiful woman has the same handicap as a rich man. The rich man can never be sure whether the woman he loves loves him or his money; and the beautiful woman can never be sure whether the man she loves loves her or her beauty. Actually, the beautiful woman is probably worse off than the rich man. He, at least, has a good chance of hanging onto his money. She learns to live in fear of the day when her physical attributes fade with age. Will her relationships fade, too?

Los Angeles marriage and family counselor Laura Schlessinger says that, like a fancy car or the right address, a beautiful woman often serves mainly to help a man stand out in society. "A lot of a man's picking out somebody who's very pretty or fits the societal model of perfection doesn't really mean that he's sexually or emotionally turned onto her at all, but that he's walking around with somebody on his arm who will give him the right *image,* regardless of how he looks. Especially if he doesn't look too great himself.

"That's the 'decorative female on the arm of the middle-aged guy with a paunch routine.' Nobody notices that he's made a slob of himself because he's got this young honey [with him]."

It's true that being seen in the company of a gorgeous woman raises a man's status. Daniel Bar-Tal of Tel-Aviv University and Leonard Saxe of Boston University did two experiments to test that hypothesis.[7] They showed students photos of men and women and asked them to speculate about their personal characteristics. The students rated such categories as popularity, intelligence, income, occupation, and marital happiness. In one of the experiments, the students rated the individuals one at a time, but in the second, the researchers paired the photos into couples. Some of the partners were equally attractive or unattractive and, in other cases, one partner was noticeably more attractive.

In the couples experiment, the unattractive man "married" to a pretty woman was rated as smarter, richer, better educated, and having higher professional status than an attractive man with a beautiful wife. The researchers' explanation for these findings is that people need to explain physically unequal relationships in some way. So, to compensate for the husband's homeliness, they imagined that he had many other qualities to offer his pretty wife. Interestingly, however, the status of a homely woman with an attractive husband was not improved at all by her husband's looks.

Evidently a woman's beauty blinds others to her real self, but a man's does not. While the beautiful woman is admired and envied, the price she pays for that attention is her individuality.

PARADOX: *Physical beauty is the most important attribute of a woman. But vanity and narcissism are sins.*

We females seem to receive these two conflicting messages from the time we're in the cradle. On the one hand we're told, "Make yourself as attractive as possible so that you can catch a husband to take care of you." On the other hand we may be called vain and narcissistic if we spend too much time and energy on making ourselves attractive. Confusion reigns. Because we can't find the appropriate path between these two poles, many of us go too far in one direction or the other, often with disastrous results. No matter which route we choose, we're likely to feel that it's the wrong one.

Gayle is a good example of a woman who bought the idea that her physical beauty was enough. "I always got lots of strokes for being pretty. But now I'm close to forty and I'm having to face the fact that looks are largely all I developed. I'm having to develop other things in myself now." As she gets older, her appearance is no longer winning her the attention it once did, and Gayle often feels disoriented and afraid.

A hazel-eyed redhead, Gayle at thirty-nine is still very attractive, but her looks are fading. She thought that her beauty was all she would ever need. "Without my hair done and without makeup, I always felt ugly. My eyes are very pale without makeup. With everything done right, though, I always got lots of attention for being pretty. But what's happening to me now is that I can't look like I want to anymore."

Approaching forty has been very frightening for Gayle, who grew up in a lower middle class family on the East Coast. "I get very scared sometimes," she admits. "I think, 'What am I going to do?' Sometimes I think that I've got to go out and get some new clothes, I've got to do something about my looks. That whole overwhelming feeling comes over me. . . ."

This emphasis on looks was ingrained early in life. The only redhead among five sisters, Gayle was considered the prettiest. Often sisters fall into different roles, which they jealously play out well into adulthood. One sister might be the smart one, another the personality, another the troublemaker. Gayle's early role stuck. As the best-looking sister, she was favored by both her parents, particularly her father. He would show her off to his friends, have her perform for them, constantly comment on how pretty she was.

School was made easier, too. "I feel that I was favored by my teachers because I was pretty. I was often chosen to give an introductory speech for a teacher, something like that, because of my looks more than anything else. And I think that, because I felt doted upon, I actually did better."

Gayle's perception that good-looking children are favored is borne out by research. Studies have shown that teachers are more likely to give a high grade to an attractive child than to one who does equal work but is unattractive. Also teachers tend to excuse a transgression by a beautiful child, yet find fault with a plain child for precisely the same behavior. Other children tend to prefer attractive playmates and to dislike unattractive ones.

An attractive child who is thus favored by her parents, teachers, and playmates learns that her beauty is the most important asset she has. She also learns that she doesn't have to try very hard to excel. If Gayle as a child, for example, wrote a C-quality theme and earned an A for it from an adoring teacher, she was robbed of her motivation to improve her writing ability. It became too easy to get by on just a smile.

The way her parents and teachers responded to her good looks was nothing, Gayle eventually learned, compared to the way men did. Getting what she wanted from men by being beautiful and charming was a snap for her. When she was eighteen she decided to escape from an increasingly oppressive homelife and legitimize her sex life. So she married a man who valued her largely for her beauty. Choosing a husband from among her boyfriends, after all, was much easier than going to college or working. The marriage lasted a little over two years.

Without a husband to support her, Gayle had to find a job, which was made easier by her looks. She became a secretary, a real asset to her company because she was so decorative. Over the years, however, Gayle has realized that being a secretary is, in many ways, simply an extension of the stereotypical feminine role: "You have to be obedient to men, charming, and passive . . . and it helps a lot if you're good-looking." She says that she "really loved the work itself. My skills were quite good. But I did not like the position it put me in."

At twenty-two, Gayle married again, this time to a man older than she who supported her very comfortably. They had two daughters, but the marriage floundered after eleven years. Suddenly she was in her thirties, twice divorced, and watching the mirror fearfully as the first signs of age crept into her face.

Luckily, Gayle is an intelligent woman who realized that she had to do something about the direction her life was taking. Her first move was to enter psychotherapy, which turned out to be a seven-year process. "I've just started to grow up and face some things [about myself] and take some responsibility in the last four or five years," she admits. "I'm more able to feel some love for myself now."

As a result of learning to value herself for qualities other than her appearance, Gayle decided to change professions. She started training as a physical therapist so that she could leave her submissive secretary role behind.

Finally, she's working on a new and more honest way to relate to the men in her life. "But I see that, for the most part, I still deal with men in a way that focuses on the way I look and being charming, and I'm disturbed about it." Changing a lifetime's behavior patterns isn't easy.

Gayle's major regret is the necessity for making these changes *now,* as her fortieth birthday approaches. It all would have been so much easier twenty years ago.

If being too narcissistic is harmful, however, being unconcerned with beauty can be equally detrimental. Annette has learned that the hard way. Unlike Gayle, Annette was taught by a Victorian mother that primping was sinful, so she developed other aspects of herself instead of her appearance. Now, at fifty-four, she's unemployed and can't seem to find another job in her field. The main problem, she's decided, is the way she looks.

Annette, who grew up in a large New England city and later moved to the West Coast, has close to twenty years' experience as a media buyer for advertising agencies. She's very good at what she does, but the problem is that nobody's hiring her to do it anymore. She's very depressed about that.

Unfortunately, Annette *looks* depressed. When we first met, she was dressed in blue jeans, a T-shirt, a lightweight poplin jacket, and tennis shoes. At least thirty pounds overweight, Barbara has not learned to dress her large physique attractively. She wears no makeup and her hair, cut in a utilitarian style, is turning from light brown to gray. She has an open, expressive face.

In a housedress, Annette would seem at home baking in an Iowa farm kitchen. There's nothing wrong with that—for an Iowa *farm woman.* But, as Annette is finding out, her style isn't appealing to a San Francisco ad agency.

"I was a victim," Annette says bluntly of the way in which she lost her last advertising job. "I had just hired and trained a good-looking young fellow and suddenly the agency I worked for said that they had to cut back on staff. So they let me go and gave my job to the guy I'd trained." That was three years ago.

For about six months, Annette applied for every job for which she was qualified, but she didn't get hired. It didn't take her long to figure out what was wrong. "I remember one agency. I had talked to the woman in charge on the phone and she said, 'Come on in.' It sounded as though my qualifications were just what they needed. I remember the woman came out into the lobby to take me into her office and I could see this change in her face immediately. When she saw me, her face just fell. By the time we got back to her office, she had nothing to say to me."

Annette blames her lack of employment on her age, and she's probably partially right. But there may be something more here, too. She looks fifty-four, but not a *stylish* fifty-four. She's a large woman, but she's not a *stylish* large woman. Advertising is a youth-oriented, stylish profession, particularly in California.

Just after she lost her job, Annette began to gain weight. "I've just gotten progressively heavier. It gets to be a factor in your life. You're heavy and you think everyone looks at you and notices you're heavy and you're never going to get anywhere." So, to make herself feel less depressed, she eats.

Annette's been supporting herself by doing clerical work for a temporary employment agency, work she dislikes and that pays much less than she earned as a media buyer. She's reached the point where she doesn't want to face another advertising agency interview. The rejection is too hard to take.

Like Gayle, Annette learned her lessons about beauty at an early age. Annette's early memories about looks center mainly on her mother. "She dominated the household. My mother did not believe in having us dressed up. We did not have clothes, other than our school uniforms."

Annette and her two sisters attended a strict Catholic school that supported their mothers' old-fashioned ideas about appearance. "Having any ego or pride was sinful. If anyone ever gave one of us a compliment, my mother would tell them, 'No, that's not true. She's not really that way at all.' She would tell them how bad we were."

After more than fifty years, Annette's voice still registers anger and bitterness: "We were not given a lot of confidence in ourselves as we grew up." Among the things about which Annette and her sisters did not gain confidence was their physical appearance.

Annette left home at twenty-four and took a job at a radio station. At that age she was an attractive young woman.

Despite leaving home, Annette was very traditional. Her first love affair was furtive. She fell in love with a divorced man so, of course, she couldn't marry him. "For a Catholic in those days, divorce was a big deal. My family would not have understood." So she kept her love life and her family separate. Her parents never even knew she had a boyfriend. She kept up appearances—in the way she'd been taught.

Annette has never married, although she would still like to find a husband. "We're late bloomers," she says with a gentle smile. One of her sisters was married for the first time, to a widower, when she was forty-six.

The painful lesson Annette is learning at fifty-four is that looks *do* count after all. Recognizing that fact is less narcissistic than realistic. A certain amount of conformity in physical appearance is a requirement if we have to depend upon others for our livelihood. We all have to be cognizant of how others perceive us. If a prospective employer interviews a depressed and dowdy middle-aged woman, he or she probably won't be impressed, no matter what the woman's qualifications are. It shouldn't be that way, perhaps, but it is.

So, like Gayle, Annette is trying to change both herself and her goals. Agency work might be too youth-oriented a profession for her, she's decided. Still, she could be a consultant. "Sometimes maturity is respected in a consultant." And she's writing. She's won several prizes for her creative efforts.

As for herself, Annette has vowed to pay more attention to how she looks. "I realize that I've just let myself go physically. Even as a consultant, I know that I'll have to go in looking good." She's starting to lose that extra weight. She's bought a couple of new dresses, a size too small, as an incentive to diet. She's trying to find a good hairdresser as well as an expert to teach her how to use makeup.

Perhaps most important, Annette is learning to feel good about herself again. She needs to raise her self-esteem so that she exudes confidence, and for women, that often goes hand in hand with feeling we are physically attractive.

Since Annette already had developed other qualities—her professional abilities, her friendship skills, her independence—she has a good start on becoming happy. For Annette as for Gayle, it would have been a lot easier to make these changes at nineteen or twenty, but that doesn't mean that they can't be made. Willing to discover a part of herself that's long been ignored, Annette figures she's still got a fighting chance at fifty-four.

We've often been told, and would like to believe, that it's what's inside of us that counts. That's not the whole truth. What's on the outside counts, too.

Unless she lives alone on a remote island, being beautiful has real consequences for a woman, and so does *not* being beautiful. Perhaps the one indisputable fact in the vast supply of information and opinion about beauty is that people respond to us, at least in part, according to the way we look. They make assumptions about us, whether they're correct or incorrect, based upon our appearance. And they act upon those assumptions.

Our physical appearance can attract or repel people. It might give us unfair advantages in life, or unfair disadvantages. It could enhance our other personal qualities or blind people to them.

Yet our looks, in a basic way, have very little to do with *who we really are.*

Physical appearance is so important, in one sense, and so unimportant, in another, that it's not surprising that most of us experience ambivalent feelings about it. The truth is, our entire society is ambivalent about beauty. We can't decide whether beauty is good or evil, powerful or weak, an advantage or a disadvantage, safe or dangerous.

We must recognize society's ambivalence about attractiveness before we can begin to resolve our own mixed feelings. We must try to discover how and when we formed our own ideas about beauty and about our own physical appearance. Once we examine the issue carefully and understand it fully, we can begin to put it into perspective for ourselves. Then we'll be well on the way to feeling, and being, truly beautiful—in the most complete sense.

5

BEAUTIFUL BABIES

When a boy baby is born, visitors to the hospital nursery are likely to comment: "What a bruiser!" "You can hear his cry on the next floor!" "What a tough little fellow!" Words of strength, hardiness, power, aggressiveness. If the baby is a girl, the comments more likely center around her looks: "What a beautiful baby!" "She certainly is a charmer!" "She'll be a real heartbreaker someday!"

One study of parental reactions to their own newborn babies showed that before the babies were a full day old, the parents perceived them as having sex-typed personalities.[1] Fathers, in particular, found differences between sons and daughters. The daughters were described as "softer, finer-featured, more awkward, more inattentive, weaker and more delicate" while the sons were seen as "firmer, larger-featured, better-coordinated, more alert, stronger and hardier." In fact, according to hospital records, the male and female babies were virtually the same in terms of length, weight, and general activity level. The traits that the parents perceived in their infants were the ones that they *expected* to see, not the traits that the babies actually possessed. Already the girls were considered more delicate and decorative.

Clothing made for infants, too, reinforces the idea that female babies are supposed to be attractive, while male babies are supposed to be active. When my son was born in 1970, the outfits available for him were rather limited, mainly miniatures of clothing that an adult male would wear: baseball suits, football uniforms, denim coveralls, sailor suits. Action was emphasized, as though the "little man" were expected to leap out of his bassinet to field a grounder.

The clothing available for girl babies is quite different. First of all, there's a much wider selection available. Go into any children's clothing store and you'll notice that the section set aside for girls' clothes is at least double the size of the department for boys' clothes. The baby outfits for girls are mainly "feminine," featuring pastel colors, particularly pink, and trimmed with ruffles, lace, ribbons, or eyelet. No kid is expected to play baseball in those getups!

We might like to think that things have changed over the past decade, but they haven't. In fact, a new mother recently wrote to the *Los Angeles Times* editorial page to bemoan the fact that it was so difficult for her to find clothing for her infant son.[2] She told of leaving the hospital with her two-day-old son and having him mistaken for a girl "based solely on the white shawl edged with a ruffle my baby was wrapped in." She cited this experience as "my first inkling that apparently society feels women [who] give birth to females have baby girls while those of us delivered of a male have little men."

My mother felt the same chagrin when my brother was born more than thirty years ago. He was a particularly beautiful baby, round-faced and rosy-cheeked, and people continually told my mother that her "little girl" was adorable, even though she dressed him in blue. "As a baby, Ken was much too pretty to be a boy," she says.

The mothers of female babies who are born without enough hair to hold a bow or who are not particularly pretty feel just as much embarrassment, perhaps more, if their babies are mistaken for boys. In fact, a girl baby loses a great deal of her value in our society if she is not beautiful. In the late sixties, a friend of mine served as a foster mother for newborn babies who were awaiting adoption. One of the infants for whom she cared was Renee, who had a birthmark on the back of her head. Little Renee was a strawberry blonde, and the birthmark was visible beneath her thin hair. Of course, that was clearly a temporary situation. As soon as she had a full head of hair, Renee's birthmark would be totally covered. In those days, healthy adoptable babies had not yet become scarce, so adoptive parents could be pretty choosy. And, when it came to Heather, they certainly were. Because she was a girl, and because she was not a beautiful girl, Renee remained in foster care for several months longer than the average foster child. More than one set of prospective adoptive parents took a look at her and decided to wait a little longer. Several parents didn't even bother to see her when they heard about her "defect."

In part, of course, this attitude simply reflects a generally negative reaction toward the female sex. Females are still viewed as decorative creatures whose major purpose is to become mothers (preferably of male children). Males, on the other hand, have a variety of purposes in life. Feminist writer Letty Cottin Pogrebin cites several surveys showing that both men and women still greatly prefer sons over daughters.[3] If a couple has only one child, according to one study, over 90 percent of the men and over 66 percent of the women prefer a male. For a firstborn, 80 percent of the couples want a son. For a three-child family, most couples prefer two boys and a girl over two girls and a boy.

This preference for sons made some sense, perhaps, years ago, when families needed boys to help with the farm labor or to run the family business. Also, of course, sons carried on the family name and could inherit property in the days when females had minimal legal rights. Today, it's discouraging that the desire for boys over girls has endured although few of the original reasons for it exist.

In this kind of atmosphere, giving birth to a daughter is often a major disappointment. Giving birth to a daughter who doesn't even live up to the expectation that she be beautiful can be considered a disaster. With the social conditioning common in our culture, it doesn't take very long for a female baby to absorb the idea that she belongs to the second-class sex. If she's pretty, at least her devaluation may stop there. If she's not, she may soon feel that she's even more of a failure.

Dr. Alice Baumgartner and her colleagues at the Institute for Equality in Education at the University of Colorado recently asked two thousand children how they thought their lives would be different if they woke up tomorrow and discovered that they had changed to the opposite sex.[4] Their answers showed that both sexes hold females in contempt. Many girls said that, if they were boys, they would be better off financially and would enjoy higher social status. They also felt that they would have more freedom and less responsibility. One girl said, "If I were a boy, my father might have loved me more."

For the girls, changing their sex might be an improvement. The boys didn't agree. They felt that if they had to be girls, they'd have to be "beautiful and know how to put on makeup and dress well." One boy said, "No one would be interested in my brain."

The message is clear: Females are prettier than males, but males are more desirable. If children don't get that message from their own parents, they'll surely get it from other sources—relatives, peers, school, television—at an early age.

The value of good looks for girls is constantly reinforced in a variety of ways. For instance, Ross D. Parke, Ph.D., professor of psychology at the University of Illinois, has found in his research that "fathers treat attractive and unattractive babies differently even in the newborn period. Fathers stimulate attractive infants more than less attractive infants. They touch, kiss, and move highly attractive infants more frequently."[5] Dr. Parke also points out that fathers pay more attention to babies who have a calm and even temperament. However, "fathers are more willing to persist in their interaction with difficult boy babies than with difficult girls."

So, a girl baby's chances of attracting her father's attention are clearly much better if she's lovely and docile.

The strongest influence on a child during the early years is clearly the parents, and, of course, different parents have different values. Los Angeles clinical psychologist J. Michael Doyle, Ph.D., says, "A child's behavior is molded according to whatever the parents' standards are, what is valued, what is appreciated." Much of the parents' value system is communicated through direct rewards to the child, Dr. Doyle says. "Girls tend to be talked about as, 'Oh, what a cute little girl; isn't she pretty?' Girls tend to be dressed up more. They get a direct message, 'This is why we value you.' "

A boy, on the other hand, according to Dr. Doyle, tends to be valued more for being able to climb up the slide or for exhibiting his physical strength or personality, or, later, for achieving good grades. A boy is valued for his accomplishments, generally in terms of his physical abilities and intelligence, while a girl is valued for something over which she has no control, her appearance. And, Dr. Doyle comments, herein lies one of the most damaging lessons little girls learn when they are valued mainly for their beauty: "Looks are nothing a child does or learns. They're something that is just there. So the view of the world that a girl soon learns, if looks are what's emphasized, is that people get ahead by luck. She doesn't have to *do* anything." If taking action and accomplishing goals bring a girl less attention than her looks, she soon learns that there's little sense in setting goals. She does not rule her own life, fate does.

Mother is the earliest influence on each of us. She gives us life, feeds us, is probably responsible for the largest part of our care when we are small and helpless. Mother is our first love because our very existence depends upon her. Mothers often teach us our first lessons in the importance of physical appearance for females. They dress us in those frilly fashions that shouldn't be soiled, and they hold us up for Daddy's approval and attention. Many of us learned early that the *only* attention we got from Daddy was when we were clean and pretty. If our diapers needed changing, or we were covered with the remains of a teething biscuit, we were quickly handed back to Mom.

Our mothers exhibit primping behavior, too. We observe that Daddy pays more attention to Mommy when she's taken the trouble to improve her appearance. As little girls, the way we learn to disconnect from our mothers, to become heterosexual creatures, is by falling in love with our fathers. Known as the Electra complex, this childhood behavior is the female counterpart of the Oedipus complex characteristic of little boys. According to traditional psychoanalytic theory, all human beings are seduced into heterosexuality when, as small children, they fall in love with the parent of the opposite sex, an attachment that later becomes inappropriate and must be resolved. The traditional psychoanalytic view of this, Dr. Doyle explains, is that a girl tries to become like her mother so that she attracts her father. So she pays particular attention to what attracts Dad to Mom.

Elena Gianini Belotti, director of a Montessori training center in Italy and author of *What Are Little Girls Made Of?*, mentions that girls begin behavior that is imitative of their mothers at an early age, probably under the age of two.[6] She writes of a typical child, Laura, previously a tomboy, whose behavior began to change markedly at the age of twenty-two months: ". . . she now began to show certain mannerisms considered typical of girls. She would sit in front of the mirror to comb her hair, and whereas previously she had often brushed her hair energetically . . . she now began to mimic an expression of complacency such as she had evidently seen used by her mother. . . . She would raise her eyebrows, bat her eyelids, smile at herself, look at herself in side-view, and bring her face nearer to and further from the mirror so as to see herself better. Some time later she arrived at the nursery with her nails painted and showed them to everybody with great pride. She became more affected. She began to want people to notice her shoes and clothes."

Laura's behavior also began to change in other ways. Earlier she had been quick to defend herself physically if attacked by another child. She now became passive and tearful. "She became less active, less daring, calmer and more apathetic and melancholy. There it was: she had become a little girl." The first sign of Laura's "taming" into "femininity" was her concern with how she looked.

Evidently Laura's mother did more than merely display primping behavior to her daughter. If she polished Laura's fingernails, the mother probably spent considerable time teaching the child that her appearance was important. Many mothers take pride in having pretty daughters; their own sense of identity is enhanced when people compliment their children. What the child wants, or whether this message is helpful to the child is often not considered.

Leslie, who grew up in the Deep South, had such a mother. "I was an only child and my mother was the oldest of eight, so she pampered me a lot. She sewed my clothes so that I could be the prettiest little girl on the block," Leslie says. "I remember being very uncomfortable with all the attention I received. I would go out with a pretty little pinafore on and I would smear dirt all over it so that I would look like all the other children. I was really embarrassed by being pretty."

When she came home wearing that dirty pinafore, however, Leslie had to face her mother's anger and a lecture on the advantages of being beautiful.

Gayle, the woman who admits that she got by mainly on her looks and now, at thirty-nine, is having to develop other qualities, also had a mother who taught her that being beautiful was the most important attribute of a female. In the evenings, her mother would line up all five daughters on the living room sofa, Gayle recalls. "She'd sit on the arm of the sofa and all of us would sit with our curlers in our laps. We'd move down one at a time and she'd curl our hair every night." The sisters slept wearing the uncomfortable curlers. If they suffered interrupted sleep because of the discomfort, that was considered a small price to pay for beauty.

Gayle recalls that she came close to rebellion against this routine some years later. "I have a memory when I was about twelve. I went through a phase where I would sit up in bed in the middle of the night, in a sleep state, and take out every one of those curlers. By the time I'd done that, though, I'd be awake, realize what I had done and sit there and recurl my hair." Today, Gayle says with a laugh, "It's not lost on me what that [her subconscious motivation] was all about. I wish I had left the curlers out at least once. I would have had a better night's sleep. And I would have found out that there *is* life on the other side of perfect hair."

Even mothers who try not to give their daughters a message that beautiful is best may convey the idea that looks are very important. I remember that my hair became an issue between my mother and me, too, but in a different way. When I was a small child, my mother would braid my sister's and my hair every morning. It was important to her that we look *neat* more than we look pretty. But somewhere—perhaps from the movies, from fairy tales, from magazines, from my playmates, from other relatives—I got the idea that I would look better if my long hair were allowed to hang freely. I hated those braids. Despite my pleas, my mother would not budge. In her opinion, I would look unkempt with my hair loose. The lesson I learned from this conflict was a subtle one: that my appearance was very, very important. That message became clear to me even though I was being taught to value neatness rather than beauty.

Some mothers give us very confusing messages about beauty, quite possibly without meaning to. Susan remembers getting many of those from her mother as she was growing up. Susan was always overweight as a child, and "my mother would comment on that a lot. Both my parents thought that I was pretty, but too heavy." Yet, she insists, "there's no question that I was overfed constantly as a child.

"I remember when I was real little, before I was even in school. My mother and I would walk to pick up my brother from school at three o'clock and we'd stop in a candy store afterwards. She would order chocolate malteds for both of us—great big silver containers, four glasses of malt—and we'd sit there and eat them with a big pretzel. That would be a mid-afternoon snack, to stave off starvation until dinnertime."

Susan admits to having a sweet tooth, even today. That, too, had its origins in her childhood. "Someone would give my mother a box of candy and she would hide it. It's a standing joke in my family that I can smell candy at a hundred paces. She could hide that candy anywhere in the house and I would find it. Then company would come over and she'd say, 'Gee, let me get out that box of candy.' And it would be all wrappers."

The effect of being told that she was too fat while she was being fed chocolate malteds and dinners dripping in gravy confused Susan. As an adult, she's still extremely sensitive about her weight, although she's much slimmer now than she was as a girl. When her own daughter was born, she made a concerted effort not to overfeed her. "When I was pregnant with my daughter, I went to interview pediatricians, to choose one. I had one main question for them: 'Do you believe in fat children?' If they did, I turned around and walked out."

Because she so vividly remembers her own unhappiness as a fat child, Susan was determined not to let her daughter become overweight. "I used to give her strained carrots for dessert when she was a baby. I figured *she* didn't know that carrots weren't dessert." Nevertheless, because she felt so bad about her own childhood appearance, Susan is teaching her daughter that looks are important and, specifically, that being overweight is a terrible state for a girl.

Susan still is angry about her mother's contribution to the weight problem that has plagued her all her life. "A couple of years back, a daughter of one of my mother's friends said that she had always resented her mother's working. My mother, having heard this, asked me if I had resented her working. I said, 'Not at all. I resented you because you made me fat.' My mother doesn't believe that she did that. I'm not quite sure *how* she doesn't believe that. She doesn't see a cause and effect relationship between being taught to eat a lot and staying fat."

Our mothers strongly influence how we feel about our looks and what we do to make ourselves look different or better. However, their influence may well be significantly less important than our fathers'. Again, traditional psychoanalytic theory is that we learn to be heterosexual by falling in love with our fathers. Daddy is the first man we know and he becomes our model for relationships with all other men in our lives. What Daddy wants in a woman is what we strive to become.

Signe Hammer, author of *Passionate Attachments: Fathers and Daughters in America Today,* writes that boys learn to *become* Daddy while girls learn to *attract* him.[7] In most cases, we do not engage in a rivalry for power with our fathers, as our brothers might. We seek to please him. So, if what Daddy wants in a female is beauty and pliability, that's what we learn to offer.

As we've seen, fathers tend to pay more attention to daughters who are good-looking, even when they are infants. And they also tend to regard their young daughters largely in terms of their sexuality and their attractiveness. Stanford University psychology professors Eleanor Emmons Maccoby, Ph.D., and Carol Nagy Jacklin, Ph.D., authors of *The Psychology of Sex Differences,* say that "a father's reactions are important in developing the femininity of his daughter. There are certain subtle ways in which he shows interest in and appreciation of his daughter's femininity."[8] They cite a study in which fathers were asked to describe the behavior of their two- and three-year-old daughters. "Here are some of the things that fathers said about their little daughters: 'A bit of a flirt, arch and playful with people, a pretended coyness.' 'Soft and cuddly and loving. She cuddles and flatters in subtle ways.' 'I notice her coyness and flirting, "come up and see me sometime" approach. She loves to cuddle. She's going to be sexy—I get my wife annoyed when I say this.' Ten out of twenty fathers described their daughters in similar terms."

Such comments may well characterize the children's behavior, but they also reflect the fathers' perceptions. Drs. Maccoby and Jacklin conclude: "The point of interest here is that the fathers appeared to enjoy being flirted with by their daughters; furthermore, the mothers . . . reported instances in which their husbands had put pressure on them to dress their daughters in dresses rather than pants, to keep their hair long, etc., when the mother would not have considered it especially important for their daughters to look dainty and feminine at this young age. Fathers appear to want their daughters to fit an image of a sexually attractive female, . . . within the limits of what is appropriate for a child, and they play the masculine role vis-à-vis their daughters as well as their wives."

Such behavior, according to the psychologists, may or may

not foster rivalry between mothers and daughters, but they believe that it is a very potent force in the child's development of the kind of behavior that her father defines as "feminine."

Signe Hammer says that fathers try to turn their daughters into an ideal of womanhood, which generally combines beauty and sexuality with passivity. She feels that many fathers give their daughters this message: "Smile for me. . . . Be pretty, entertain and nourish and satisfy me; sympathize. But don't grow up to become a threatening woman like my mother, or like yours. Remain innocent and controllable."

Marriage and family counselor Laura Schlessinger agrees. "Daddies can play little games [of power and control] with their daughters that they wouldn't dare to do with wives, who'd tell them to kiss off and drop dead. With little girls, Dad's the big power."

His ideal little woman is one who looks gorgeous and gives him no flak. Yet, as a lesson in how to relate to men when she grows up, this behavior doesn't benefit his daughter. Such a daughter may well relate to all men—lovers, husbands, teachers, employers—as she does to her father, seductively.

Children, Dr. Schlessinger says, "are not independent creatures and they don't have access to other ways" of behaving, beyond the ones their parents teach them. They learn that being seductive with Daddy gets them what they want.

Often, Dr. Schlessinger says, a daughter might not only earn herself more of Daddy's attention but get herself out of trouble by using seductive behavior with him. If she hasn't done her homework, for instance, her father might threaten punishment. If she argues with him or is belligerent, he's likely to come down hard on her. After all, he has the power. But, if she acts seductively and says, "Oh, Daddy, I just didn't have the time. Can *you* help me with it?" she flatters him and diverts him from punishing her.

According to Hammer, girls learn to get what they want

by being manipulative and seductive with their fathers. "If he is an indulgent Daddy, we feel our power in 'seducing' him into giving us what we want. The first time Daddy, with an indulgent smile, agrees to buy us the toy or dress that Mother said we couldn't have, we sense the beginning of a female power that, we are taught, can take us a long way." She points out that daughters can relate to fathers and the power those fathers possess in ways that sons cannot. The sons' "job is to learn how to *become* this power, this authority. But our job is to seduce it, and to be seduced by it."

This way of relating to men is undoubtedly not the most constructive one to pursue once we're adults, but while we're still little girls, being noticed and indulged by Daddy because we're pretty and entertaining and flattering to his ego can seem quite wonderful. We are impressed by how easily this kind of behavior gets us what we want. Some fathers can't relate to their daughters in any other way.

As a rather extreme example of this fact, Gayle had a father who not only taught her that her role in life was to be beautiful and charming, he reinforced that message by making life seem quite dangerous whenever she wasn't beautiful and charming enough.

"I can remember when I was a child, my father would call home from the neighborhood bar, where he would be with his friends, and say, 'Send Gayle up here. I want to show her off,' " Gayle says. A man with a serious drinking problem, Gayle's father tended to spend a lot of time in that bar.

"He'd often come home drunk with a couple of his friends on a Friday or Saturday night and say, 'Wake Gayle up,' " she recalls. "He would want me to come out and sing and entertain for his friends." Gayle was the only one of his five daughters subjected to this routine. She was the prettiest, and, therefore, her father's favorite. In some ways, his attention made her feel special in comparison with her sisters. But it also put a great deal of pressure on her to keep the peace in a tension-filled household. "We were all afraid of my father. He was often physically abusive to my mother, although not to us. I thought that, if I could entertain him well enough, do a good enough job [of being pretty and charming], he would fall asleep and then he wouldn't hit my mother."

The message Gayle received is clear: Not only will being pretty and charming earn her a man's attention, it will keep her safe from his violent nature, which might erupt at any moment. Under these circumstances, how could any young girl dare *not* become what her father wanted her to be?

For Gayle's father, clearly a woman's beauty was evidence of her sexuality. In his daughter he could define that sexuality as innocent. In his wife, however, it became threatening. "When I look back at the pictures of my mother as a young woman, she was always dressed so nicely, and she was an attractive woman, too. She really cared about having things stylish and just right. My father was so jealous that he didn't want her to wear makeup. He didn't want her looking attractive. I think she was very frustrated about that."

A few years later, Gayle's mother finally asserted herself and "sneaked out to get a part-time job. She bought herself a few clothes, but my father went into a rage and cut them all up."

Some fathers are unable to view even their young daughters' sexuality as innocent; they feel attracted and threatened by it. Leslie, dressed by her mother in those frilly pinafores she persisted in dirtying, feels that her stepfather was one of those men. She and her mother lived with him from the time Leslie was a toddler until she was fifteen. "He would tease me about being prettier than the other girls and that would make me feel real uncomfortable," she recalls. "And, from the time I was real little, he was adamant about my never getting involved with a boy. Starting about the time I was five or six, he would sit me down and lecture me that I was never to be seen holding hands with a boy. He told me that I wouldn't be allowed to date until I was eighteen."

Leslie wasn't quite sure just what would be wrong with holding hands with a boy, but she sensed that her prettiness might instigate some kind of forbidden behavior. She often noticed little boys, but not without feeling guilty about it. One day, when she was eight, Leslie attended her cousin's school. Several of the little boys in the cousin's class wrote Leslie love notes. Instead of appreciating the innocent affection proclaimed in those notes, she "burst into tears because I was so upset by all that attention. I felt real dirty. I wanted to run and get away from it all. I felt real degraded and dirty."

Leslie says that she "could sense sexuality in the situation. I guess it was basically that I thought the boys would want to kiss me." Kissing, of course, is several steps beyond the hand-holding about which her stepfather had warned her.

After that experience, Leslie gained quite a bit of weight, which she didn't lose until puberty. She thinks that subconsciously she added the extra pounds so that there would be no chance of her attracting a boyfriend.

While her stepfather was reacting so negatively to the possibility of puppy love for Leslie, however, her mother continued to emphasize the child's appearance, dressing her in frilly clothes, and curling her hair every night. "My mother treated me like a doll. So I was being pulled in both directions at once."

Her extra weight stayed on until Leslie was in the seventh grade and had begun her menstrual period. Then the tension between her and her stepfather grew stronger. "I would notice him looking at me, so I wore loose clothing around him and made sure that I was never alone with him." There was an ugly incident at this time involving the cousin whose class Leslie had visited a few years earlier. "She had developed real early and my stepfather once fondled her breast. She confided that to me, so I was even more frightened of him after that."

She and her cousin told Leslie's mother about the sexual incident, but, Leslie says, "my mother was not ready to leave him at that time, so she made up excuses for him in her mind, that somehow my cousin had done something to attract him. She avoided the issue."

Leslie's mother was a true Southern belle, a woman who felt that she could not make it without a man. She was getting older and the one asset she felt she had to attract another husband, her beauty, was fading. So she wasn't willing to leave the husband who was supporting her without knowing which man would be next. Nevertheless, she didn't leave Leslie entirely unprotected against a potentially incestuous relationship. "After we talked to her about him, I noticed that my mother became much more protective of me. She made sure that I was never alone in the house with him. So, if she went to the supermarket in the morning, for instance, she would wake me up and take me with her."

Leslie had the intelligence to sense that her stepfather was sexually attracted to her and, thus, she didn't engage in any kind of seductive behavior with him. Had she done so, she might well have given him an excuse to turn their relationship into an incestuous one.

Most such men feel inadequate in many areas of their lives, so they turn to the least threatening of creatures, very young females, for affection. If a father has a basic sense of inadequacy, and if that father can transform his daughter into his ideal female—one who is beautiful, flattering, sexual, and totally acquiescent—incest may result. The most common age for incest to take place, by the way, is nine, well before the daughter has developed secondary sex characteristics. And well before she has become a threatening adult.

Dr. Schlessinger tells about a couple of families that she has counseled in her Los Angeles practice. "The fathers in the families had feelings of inadequacy disguised in brashness and loudness and bullying. In one family, in particular, the wife was not taking any of this and was rather brash back. And he found the kind of sweetness and seductiveness in the daughter that he did not find in his wife. These are often the beginnings of incest." She points out, however, that incestuous relationships, in the broad sense, don't always have to be sexual. "It can be a relationship in which most of the emotional, seductive, tender feelings are directed toward the little girl instead of toward the wife."

If a man is inclined toward sexual relations with his daughter, any seductive behavior on her part can be interpreted as an invitation. This often contributes to the unwarranted guilt that incest victims ultimately feel. "Men use any excuse they can find to rationalize incest," says Dr. Schlessinger. "But when kids are seductive, they don't know what they're doing. All they know is that, when they act this way, somebody treats them very nicely and shows them lots of attention. They don't understand that they're being seductive in a true sexual way, the way an adult woman would if she put on a long black dress and her best perfume."

The way our fathers treat us when we are small has a profound effect on our adult relationships with men, and upon our general self-esteem. The ideal father will reassure his daughter that she is pretty and feminine and sexually attractive; and he will also reaffirm her worth in other ways, by telling her that she is capable, intelligent, strong, independent, and so on. With the impact of the feminist movement and the increasing interest of many modern men in fathering, I think that today's children have a greatly improved chance of having that ideal father. But, when most of us were small, sex roles were prescribed and mothers were expected to do most of the child rearing. In those days, it was the rare father, indeed, who realized the impact that he would have on his daughter's life. Yet we all live with the effects of that very important early influence upon us.

Henry Biller, Ph.D., author of *Father Power*, says that research done on father-daughter relationships indicates that women who, as children, enjoyed close, positive associations with their fathers are more likely to have stable, romantic liaisons as adults.[9] A strong father-daughter relationship has also been found to relate to the daughter's later ability to achieve orgasm. "The high-orgasm women . . . recalled their fathers as having a definite set of values, being demanding, and having high expectations for them," Dr. Biller writes. "Women who rarely achieved orgasm reported their fathers as being casual, permissive and unavailable for deep involvement. They were more likely to say that they could not set up a relationship with their father either because he had died early in their lives or because of his job."

Those of us lucky enough to have fathers who made us feel competent and worthwhile undoubtedly enjoy important and valuable advantages as adults. Unfortunately, not all of us can count ourselves in that group.

Some of us may have had fathers who failed in some way to reaffirm our basic value. Perhaps they were either physically or emotionally absent from the home. Some fathers may have preferred sons and felt that daughters were not worth their attention. Others may have reassured us that we were smart or pious or responsible, but ignored our appearance and sexuality, perhaps because our more feminine attributes were too threatening for them to deal with.

Others of us had fathers who affirmed our worth *solely* in terms of our beauty and sexuality, perhaps because they felt that females are useful only as sex objects or as mothers. Those of us with that kind of father likely grew up feeling helpless and worthless without a male protector.

With a father at either extreme, we learn to feel somehow less than whole. What little girls need is a father who is able and willing to help us feel successful, not only as females, but as people.

Although our parents are the major influence upon us in our early years, they are certainly not the only influence. Another vital force in our lives is siblings. In families with more than one child, for instance, each tends to take on a specific role. Gayle is a good example. Her role was clearly that of "the pretty one." Her oldest sister, in contrast, played the role of "the rebellious one," as the only one of the five sisters who would try to oppose their father.

Sharon, an old friend of mine who has a sister, ten years older than she, remembers that when they were children, people would constantly remark upon her sister's beauty. "They'd always say that Andrea was the pretty one and that Sharon was . . . well, 'spunky' or something like that. I grew up thinking that I must be a terribly ugly girl. But now I look back and see pictures of me as a kid and *I* was good-looking, too. It's just that Andrea was gorgeous."

Not until she was over forty did Sharon finally begin to feel that she was truly attractive. Actually, the role of "the spunky one" didn't serve her too badly, either. Thinking of herself as spunky, in other words, as a sharp and competent risk-taker, helped Sharon travel around the world when she was in her twenties, and to begin law school when she was already in her late thirties, divorced, and the mother of two sons.

Undoubtedly, all children need reassurance from someone whose opinion they value that they are, indeed, physically attractive. Of course, it doesn't help to lie to a basically ugly child, yet it seems to me that there is *something* physically attractive about nearly any child, perhaps her smile or her sturdy body or her hair. And, let's face it, physical appearance is an important part of feminine sexuality. Ironically, for those of us who are average, it can be difficult to find reassurance that the way we look is, after all, passable. Almost any other part of a little girl's life has a "report card" attached to it to let her know where she stands, that she's done well. Schoolwork comes with letter grades. If a child does chores around the house to earn an allowance, the money serves as a reward. If she likes to sew or bake or sculpt or build, her creations offer proof of her talent. But, since looks are something that simply exist, not something we accomplish, we may grow up feeling unpretty unless we receive that reassurance. As psychologist J. Michael Doyle points out, too much emphasis on appearance can be harmful. Perhaps, so can too little.

Like Sharon, my friend Terri, who's forty-three now and a highly accomplished businesswoman, is a good example. Terri always felt unattractive as a child, not because anyone ever told her she was ugly, but because no one ever told her she was pretty. As an adult, she's still fighting that negative self-image on a daily basis. Even owning her own business has not erased the memory of herself formed in childhood of a plain, inadequate little girl.

With sisters, beauty is an easy reason for rivalry to occur. If one is clearly "the pretty one," the others may feel inferior even though they do well in their own chosen roles. If she has only brothers, a girl may be *forced* into the role of the pretty one.

According to Dr. Doyle, most parents differentiate fairly sharply between the way they treat their daughters and the way they treat their sons. "A girl who has a brother and who sees that he's treated differently than she is will have to come to some sort of resolution with that. There are various ways to do that, and one is to play the feminine game. That's probably easiest." So, instead of trying to compete with her brother or brothers in terms of physical abilities or accomplishments or intelligence, many little girls will fall back on the one area in which her brothers aren't able to compete with her—femininity. "If the family is one in which the mother is not a strong, independent person and her main way of valuing herself is in her appearance and her ability to attract a man," then there's even more pressure on the daughter to conform to the feminine stereotype.

Even when the daughter does accept the role of the delicate, pretty child in contrast to her brothers' roles, she can face a rocky childhood. They may resent the attention she receives as a girl and the fact that they have to compete on a different level. That's what happened to Cecily, the third and youngest child, and the only daughter, of a Chicago doctor and his wife. "My parents were always very supportive of me and told me how cute I was," Cecily says today. "My brothers, on the other hand, resented me because my parents seemed to favor me. As a result, they somehow found a weakness in me and punched into it. They kept calling me ugly, and they got the next-door neighbor kids to call me ugly, too. This went on for years and years."

Cecily realizes now that she was not really an ugly child, but at the time, she took her brothers' taunts completely to heart. "I was neither ugly nor beautiful, I guess. But I really got a complex about my looks. I think that other children can sense what makes a child feel bad, and they zero in on that. So other children sort of attacked me, too. The more that happened, the more I withdrew into myself."

As a toddler, Cecily's looks were average. But, at the age of seven, her worsening eyesight forced her to wear glasses. And "I sucked my thumb until I was twelve, so I had rather bucked teeth, too," she recalls, and adds with pain in her voice, "I was called 'four eyes' or 'bucktooth,' things like that."

Cecily's situation illustrates how the influence of peers becomes more and more important as a child grows older. "My parents always came to my defense: 'She's not ugly. How can you say that?' But they were the only ones telling me that I was *not* ugly and my peers and my brothers were telling me that I *was.* So who would I believe?"

In reaction, Cecily tried to reject the role of little girl, in which she felt she was failing, and become a boy. She wore flannel shirts and jeans and climbed trees. Even though she was younger and couldn't win, she tried to compete against her brothers in their arena. She feels that probably sparked even more resentment. "I remember telling my father, 'I wish

I'd been born a boy.' He said, 'Why? You can have babies and boys can't.' But I said, 'I don't see anything very special about that.' He couldn't kid me."

In one way, Cecily was her father's favorite, but she thinks that was only because he didn't really treat her as a person. "My dad was really outrageous. He would spank my brothers, but he would never spank me. I really do resent the fact that I was treated like a doll, a little golden doll. In a way, I was like a cute little object to him. I fought back ferociously, but he thought that was cute, too. When I would exert myself and my opinions, he would dismiss me as 'cute.' I would say, 'Hey, Daddy, *listen* to me,' but he didn't hear me. He just thought I was cute."

Also, Cecily's father would invariably take her side in her battles against her brothers, and that made things even worse among the children. "He was very militaristic with them," she recalls.

She learned specific ways to deal with him that were not available to the boys. "I would climb up on his lap and scratch his chin and he'd give me a quarter. I really learned to manipulate him and he loved it." Cecily often watched her mother use similar tactics to get what she wanted from her father. "He was crazy about her, too. If she would kind of cozy on up to him and act a little bit girlish, he would give her whatever she wanted. He loved to give us things. If we couldn't decide between four dresses, he'd say, 'Take them all.' "

Yet, even with what seemed to be the support and indulgence of her father and mother, Cecily grew up feeling ugly and rejected. She had no doubt that because she was a girl, her appearance was the most important thing about her. *That* message was clear from both camps—her parents, who told her that she was pretty and cute, on the one side, and her brothers and peers, who told her she was ugly, on the other. Because she believed that she was a failure at the most important thing a female can have—beauty—she later worked her way through a series of degrading love affairs and spent many of her adult years trying to repair her damaged self-esteem.

A year or so ago, when Cecily was in her late twenties, she even wrote one of her brothers a letter to the effect that he had ruined her sex life. In part, she wrote: "I can't tell you how many men I've been to bed with because I felt ugly. It ruined a lot of my life." Her brother's reaction? "At first he was very upset and angry with me," she says, "but since then he's been treating me a lot more like an adult. I felt good about writing that letter, about letting him know what he'd done to me. I didn't really care if he responded or not."

If we don't learn the significance of beauty from our families and our peers, there are plenty of outside influences to teach us, such as the literature of childhood. Today, children have a wide variety of books with strong female heroines available to them. When we were children, things were different, and we still feel the effects of those early teachings. I remember growing up largely on fairy tales, from about the age of two until I was nine or ten. Occasionally I read a book featuring a heroine with some gumption—*Heidi* or *Little House on the Prairie,* and when I was older, I read the Nancy Drew series—but most of the books available to me at a young age were fairy tales. I spent hours escaping into their fantasy world. These traditional childhood stories convey strong values that little girls take very much to heart.

We can choose just about any fairy tale and find the theme of a beautiful young girl waiting passively for a prince to be bowled over by her beauty, marry her, and live happily ever after with her. Not one of these patient young damsels ever stuns the prince with her intelligence, her kindness, her love of children, her business sense, her sparkling wit. No, it's her *beauty* that wins him every time. Sleeping Beauty, in fact, was gorgeous enough to get her man despite her being totally comatose.

Virtually all female characters in the fairy tales fall into one of two categories—they're evil and ugly, or they're beautiful and good. Interestingly, the evil women far outnumber the heroines. In the Grimm fairy tales, Elena Gianini Belotti points out, a full 80 percent of the females are portrayed as evil. The remaining 20 percent are mainly beautiful young girls waiting for that knight on the white charger.

These stories are filled with sexual imagery, of course. Letty Cottin Pogrebin notes that at puberty, the typical young girl in a fairy tale is taken out of action before her sexual power can be explored. She requires a handsome prince-husband to save her, and to awaken her sexuality in the proper, married state. "So, when Rapunzel turns twelve, she is imprisoned in a tower, her hair (her childhood strength, her rope to freedom) cut off," Pogrebin says. "Snow White eats the red apple (menstruation? sexual knowledge?) but before she can lose her innocence, she's out cold. Sleeping Beauty pricks her finger and before the (menstrual) blood is dry, she's asleep, too. For a girl coming out of childhood, passive is good but catatonic is better." And beautiful, of course, is definitely required.

The female in the fairy tale is actually an attractive possession, and her pure and innocent sexuality must not be damaged in any way before she can be transferred from her father to her husband.

These stories often provide a distorted view of life, says UCLA associate professor of English Karen Rowe, who specializes in fairy tales and folklore. "What I think is problematic for the twentieth century reader of the popular tales is that no provision is made for activity on the part of the heroine. It's all rescue, all passivity.[10]

"What that communicates to a female child is that it's

never by your own will or action that you overcome a problem. It's [only] through intervention on your behalf by some other figure. That undercuts any sense of growth and leads to a cultural emphasis on female dependency, which I think is very destructive."

Not only is a girl taught by these tales that she cannot act for herself, she's taught that, unless she's beautiful, she won't be able to attract a handsome prince.

The toys and playthings available for children often reinforce the idea that beauty is a major concern. Ironically, the toys available for little girls include some that are more progressive and others that are more regressive than those we had.

Fortunately, today's little girls can play with doctor kits as well as nurse kits, with electronic games as well as baking sets, with toy musical instruments as well as toy vacuum cleaners. Many toys have become unisex.

Still, there are many toys that always have been marketed largely for girls. And those are the ones that emphasize physical appearance.

Dolls are an obvious example. Most of us played with them when we were kids, and I remember that one of the most popular was the doll that could be dressed in a variety of different, fashionable outfits. Paper dolls with their many wardrobe changes were similarly important to us. In the years since my childhood, the dolls available to little girls have become far more sophisticated, and in becoming so, they may well emphasize the significance of beauty to a new extreme. Some of the new dolls, for instance, even teach a child to style and set hair. Even the quarter-century-old Barbie doll has become more beauty conscious. In fact, Barbie's inventor, Bill Barton, feels that today's Barbie simply has gone too far in that direction. Recently, Barton, who designed the famous doll in 1958, naming it after his daughter, expressed concern about the thin, almost undernourished body and sexy appearance of the latest Barbie. "I think it has had a negative effect on some girls. Some girls look in the mirror when they're teenagers and are disappointed when they don't see Barbie."[11]

Like playing with dolls, dressing up in adult clothing is another pastime that little girls have probably always enjoyed. It's a way of playing grown-up, of trying out behavior the child considers mature. As long as it remains a game, it's perfectly normal. Perhaps it becomes abnormal when miniature adult clothes, many of which are quite overtly sexual, are manufactured in children's sizes as they often are today.

As a child growing up in the fifties, I remember playing with makeup to a small degree. Candy lipstick was very popular. Rubbing the gooey stuff on my lips made me feel very grown-up, and, besides, it tasted good. Compared to what's available for today's little girls, however, candy lipstick was pretty tame stuff. Now, young girls have complete makeup kits, lighted makeup mirrors, toy wigs, nail polish. These beauty aids are marketed for children as young as three, and they cost as much as twenty-five dollars.

This emphasis on physical appearance at such an early age is very harmful to children, according to Sam Janus, Ph.D., a New York City psychotherapist and associate clinical professor of psychiatry at New York Medical College. "The problem is, when you give these makeup kits at three, by eight they want the real thing. It encourages them to look at their bodies as sex objects."[12]

Dr. Janus thinks that our society is sexualizing childhood to an extreme degree these days. He cites sexy jeans ads featuring twelve-year-old models, the increasing number of pubescent prostitutes, and the proliferation of child pornography as evidence of his thesis.

Perhaps a less visible kind of evidence is the lack of self-esteem displayed by girls who are reared to think that their beauty, their sexuality, is the most important part of themselves. Certainly the toys and playthings available to them reinforce this damaging idea.

After the home, school is probably the second most important arena in which young girls learn that beautiful is better. For instance, a study conducted by psychologists Ellen Berscheid, Elaine Walster, and Margaret Clifford shows that teachers have higher academic expectations of attractive children than of unattractive ones.[13] The psychologists asked four hundred fifth-grade teachers to examine student report cards and draw some conclusions about each student. Each report card included a photograph of a child, either one of six boys and girls judged to be attractive, or one of six boys and girls judged to be unattractive. As the researchers predicted, the teachers assumed that the good-looking boy or girl who had a higher I.Q., would be more likely to attend college, and had parents interested in his or her education. The teachers also hypothesized that the better-looking children related better to their classmates than did the less attractive students.

In another study, by psychologist Karen Dion, subjects were asked to evaluate misbehavior by children whose photographs they were shown.[14] As Dion expected, they assumed that a misdeed by a pretty child was an isolated incident, while the same misdeed by an unattractive child was considered typical behavior for that child. A similar study by Leonard Berkowitz and Ann Frodi required that subjects select appropriate discipline for a ten-year-old girl.[15] If the girl was attractive, the discipline selected for her was less severe than that chosen for the unattractive girl.

Berscheid and Walster conclude that "in cases in which there is some question about who started the classroom disturbance, who broke the vase, or who stole the money (and with children it always seems that there is the question of *who did it?*) adults are likely to identify an unattractive child as the culprit. . . . Thus, if an unattractive child protests his innocence, his pleas may fall on deaf ears. The long march to the principal's office starts early, and physical unattractiveness may be a silent companion for the marcher."

Findings such as those of Berscheid, Walster, Clifford,

Dion, Berkowitz, and Frodi are particularly important when we consider that often adults' expectations of children become self-fulfilling prophecies. Some of us may well remember being treated either better or worse than our classmates by a grammar school teacher and not knowing why. In many cases, the cause was the teacher's possibly unwarranted conclusions about us, based on appearance. Certainly many of us can recall the child who was the teacher's pet. Chances are that he or she was good-looking.

If we received such favor during our formative years, we may have learned, either directly or indirectly, that our beauty was a very valuable asset. If we watched better-looking children receive extra attention and affection, we may have been taught an additional lesson in school: to feel bad about ourselves because of something over which we had no control.

Little boys, as well as little girls, experience discrimination if they are not attractive. But since so many other avenues to achievement are open to boys, like excelling in sports, it's easier for a boy to overcome any stigma attached to his looks. An unattractive boy may suffer briefly, but with effort in other directions, he still has the opportunity to form a healthy self-image.

The other kids in school help teach us the painful lesson that our looks count. Psychologist Richard Lerner of Pennsylvania State University says that children from about the age of five on tend to reject fat people, and he adds, "Very early, children recognize the implications of being ugly versus being attractive."[16]

When Berscheid and Walster questioned nursery school children, ages four to six, they found that the children preferred their more attractive classmates as friends. Being unattractive was not a big drawback for a four-year-old girl, but by the time she was six, her popularity with her peers was decidedly declining. The less attractive girls also were judged by the other children to be less independent and more fearful than their prettier classmates.

As we progress from babyhood into school age, we learn to be more and more concerned with appearance in the broadest sense of the word: our beauty (or lack of it), our clothing, our behavior, the friends we choose, indicators of our family's wealth and values. We might describe this process as acquiring a concern for "what the neighbors think."

We learn this concern from our parents, from our friends, from school, from books, from television.

It's probably easiest to see how our parents pressure us in this direction. Traditionally, many parents treat their children as extensions of themselves, and thus feel they must make sure that the rest of the world responds positively to their children. If people like us, it's virtually the same as their liking our parents. They are validated by our success.

At the extreme of parents who value beauty above all else in their daughters are those who enter their children in any of the five thousand child beauty pageants held in the United States each year. Some parents even make a hobby of taking their young daughters from contest to contest on weekends and during summer vacations, displaying them in the hope of winning a prize. Such pressure can be extremely difficult for a child, particularly if she seldom wins.

One New York psychiatrist says of these contests: "I think the parents do it for themselves. They don't respect the rights and interests of the child. I had one psychotic patient who had a history of competing in beauty contests. She couldn't take the pressure, but the pageants became the only gratification in her life."[17]

Some of these parents become truly obsessed with having their daughter officially certified as the prettiest little girl in town. The pressure they put on their children to be beautiful and charming can be bizarre. One mother of a three-year-old contestant, for instance, was observed slapping the child for crying, which made her makeup run. Another dressed her two-year-old daughter for a contest in an incongruous costume consisting of diapers and false eyelashes.

Luckily, most of us did not have parents who pushed us into the beauty trap quite that firmly. Nevertheless, females learn the benefits of beauty at a very early age. If we're told that we're beautiful as children, and we believe it, we may well feel fortunate. But we may also be learning behavior that will harm us in later life—that we should focus all our worth on an asset that fades with time. If we learn that we're not beautiful, we may well form the beginnings of an inferiority complex that will plague us for a lifetime. We may try to compensate for our lack of good looks by excelling in other areas of our lives. Yet, even if we succeed, the seeds of self-hatred may have already taken root.

Whatever we have learned about our own physical appearance and its importance, chances are that *we will leave childhood believing that a successful female is a beautiful female.* Before we reach the next, and perhaps most difficult, period of life—adolescence—we will already have begun the kind of thinking that will eventually catch us in the beauty trap.

6

BECOMING BEAUTIES

The work of adolescence, writes psychoanalyst Erik Erikson, is to determine who we are. During this time of life, we separate emotionally from our parents, and our peers become more important to us. Adolescence is a time of change, a time of rebellion, a time to form our own value system. These emotional and psychological changes are accompanied by vast, sometimes overwhelming physical changes. How we look is the external manifestation of who we are, and in adolescence, how we look changes almost daily. So coming to terms with our new physical appearance is a most important part of resolving the identity crisis that Erikson describes.

I remember some of the styles that were in fashion when I was growing up in the fifties and early sixties. We often wore full skirts with several petticoats (sometimes soaked in sugar water and dried to make them stiffer), cinch belts, and blouses. Sometimes we donned a sheath dress or occasionally a "tight" skirt (which wasn't tight at all by today's standards) with a sweater set. We scrunched our feet into pointed-toe shoes, either T-strap flats or, if we were feeling particularly grown-up, stiletto heels that poked holes in linoleum floors. Our hair, if we wore it long, was in a pageboy or pulled back in a ponytail, or, if we preferred it shorter, in a "bubble" cut. We wore makeup in moderation, usually lipstick and face powder or blusher, and occasionally mascara. We didn't want to look either too drab or too "cheap."

The particular style that each of us remembers from our own teen years—whether it's "strawberry float" saddle shoes or miniskirts, baggy jeans rolled below the knees or T-shirts worn without a bra—doesn't really matter. What's popular with teenagers seems to change from one week to the next. What doesn't change is the adolescent's need to conform. And how teenagers look is the outer symbol of their conformity, their badge of belonging to their particular group. Yet, at the same time, adolescents also have a need to assert their individuality. So conformity is at war with individuality in the adolescent mind, all part of the confusing emotional process of determining, "Who am I?"

Dr. Gerald Dabbs of New York's Payne Whitney Psychiatric Clinic outlines four factors that all normal teenagers experience and which often contribute to their typical feelings of confusion and inadequacy: [1]

1. Adolescence is a period of extreme biochemical changes, which by themselves can create depressive states.
2. Teenagers become more introspective. They view themselves supercritically, almost as if they felt a need to dislike and disapprove of what they see.
3. Human sexuality reaches a fever pitch during adolescence. Experimentation is common and guilt-producing.
4. Teens experience a period of mourning as they cut ties to their parents, who have been their source of values, of security, and of approval. Their subconscious response to this change is often as if they had experienced a death in the family.

"Adolescents feel so intensely," Dr. Dabbs says, "that they can't imagine everyone doesn't know how miserable they are."

Physical appearance is often the easiest place on which to pin these feelings of misery. "If only I had the right hair (or figure or clothes or face)," the teenager tells herself, "my life would be perfect." If she just *looked* perfect, she believes, she could *be* perfect.

Perhaps one of the main reasons why adolescents are so obsessed with the way they look is that this time of life heralds the process of sexual maturation. Girls at eleven or twelve begin to develop breasts, pubic hair appears, their hips become rounder, they experience their first menstrual period. And they begin to notice boys. A few years later, boys begin to notice them.

Since adolescence is so new, and is not yet accompanied by much in the way of emotional maturity, teenage sexual attraction is based almost completely on looks. So physical appearance becomes vital. After all, it's what will attract the opposite sex, and boys are often the most important thing in a teenage girl's life.

Largely because they want to attract boys, girls are often accused of being vain at this age. But psychologists Dr. Eleanor Emmons Maccoby and Dr. Carol Nagy Jacklin believe that both sexes are narcissistic, although in different ways.[2] "It is the boy with the most status and power (as well as a reasonable amount of good looks) who can interest the most attractive girls," they say. "Traditionally it has been the most beautiful, alluring girl who can interest the highest-status boys. When a girl dresses in an eye-catching manner, or expends a great deal of time on her hair and makeup, she is making a statement to boys about her interest in them, as well as seeking admiration for herself. Similarly when a boy 'shows off' to girls, he is signaling to them that he has status and potency; at the same time, he is certainly not free of narcissism."

This emerging sexuality can be the cause of friction between teenage girls and their parents. Although it is entirely normal, budding sexuality is threatening in a variety of ways to parents. Their reactions often make their daughters feel that there is something wrong with them, something terrible they have done in the process of growing up.

Mothers may not want to face the fact that their daughters are becoming teenagers. As they watch their daughters change—grow taller, acquire curves, become sexual—they have to acknowledge many transformations in their own lives. Researcher Natalie Shainess has shown, for instance, that many mothers react negatively to their daughters' first menstrual periods, which are, of course, symbolic evidence of womanhood.[3]

"The question of why menstruation has been such a thorny subject for mothers and daughters is not easily answered," says Signe Hammer, author of *Daughters and Mothers, Mothers and Daughters*.[4] "It heralds the time when a daughter becomes defined by her sexuality (that is, by her capacity to bear children), to which most other aspects of her personal development henceforth will be subordinated. Any mother who resents the choices she has had to make is likely to react negatively to her daughter's reaching this point."

Such a mother may also simply feel old as her daughter grows into a woman. She may notice her wrinkles and sagging skin in the mirror just as her daughter is blooming. She may feel that added age diminishes her own value.

She may feel sexually competitive with her daughter, too. Dr. Laura Schlessinger points out that a well-adjusted mother will be proud of her attractive teenage daughter, but the woman who has problems with self-esteem may react with jealousy to her child's maturing. "This kind of competition doesn't really come out of the woodwork when the daughter reaches her teens," she explains. "Generally there are seeds of it earlier—Dad may have been paying more attention to the daughter all along."

When the child develops into an attractive young woman, the mother finds a target for her own unhappiness. "My daughter's getting all this attention," she tells herself, "because she's prettier than I am." She comes to resent the attention, and her daughter, bitterly.

"The mother becomes hostile to the daughter's beauty because she's made it into a scapegoat," explains Dr. Schlessinger. "But the *real* problem is the mother's feelings about herself and her relationship with her man."

Whatever the individual reason, when mothers react negatively to their daughters' growing up, which is symbolized by the onset of menarche, daughters undoubtedly decide that something is very wrong with them. And whatever that something is concerns the way their bodies are changing.

Many mothers, instead of dreading their daughters' maturing, may actually look forward to it, so that they can relive their own lives through their offspring. "Often," says Dr. Schlessinger, "you'll have a case where the mother will support her child's being seductive so that the child can get attention that Mama didn't get as a girl. She'll live vicariously through her daughter." Having a teenage daughter might give some mothers a second chance to live through their own difficult adolescent years. This time, they tell themselves, they'll be far more successful. Unfortunately, this attitude ignores the daughter's need for independence. Of course, it also makes life terribly difficult for daughters who simply can't live up to their mothers' expectations.

When Jenny, now thirty-two, had reached adolescence, her mother, Margaret, alternated trying to live vicariously through Jenny and being competitive with her. "My mother is very much into looks," Jenny says today. "I would say that she's obsessed with the way she looks." And there was a time when she was obsessed with the way Jenny looked. Weight became an issue, for instance. Margaret dieted constantly and achieved much of her sense of identity through her ability to maintain a svelte figure. "She would get very upset if I ever gained any weight," Jenny recalls.

Jenny's mother often used her niece, Pam, who had a weight problem, as a negative example. "Pam has gained weight again and her mother is really upset about it," Margaret would say to Jenny, her voice filled with panic. "She's got to lose it!"

Margaret made Pam's weight gain sound as though she had failed her mother in a most essential way. Jenny remembers wondering whether her aunt still loved Pam even though the girl was fat. Jenny feared how her own mother would feel about her if she ever added too many pounds. The message she received from her mother was that being heavy would make her unlovable.

At the same time, Jenny could tell that her mother was congratulating herself for having a thinner daughter than her sister. The sibling rivalry that had always raged between Margaret and her sister was still going strong over the issue of their daughters' looks.

In addition to weight, clothes became an issue between Jenny and Margaret. "My mother was always taking me clothes shopping. And I just didn't care about clothes that much." The clothes Jenny selected were unusual and individual. The clothes Margaret wanted to buy for her were whatever was the latest fashion.

As Jenny grew older, she began to resent her mother's attempts to dictate the way she should look and to rebel. Achieving autonomy meant rejecting her mother's values to form her own. In doing so, Jenny rejected the idea that she should focus her life on the way she looked. In fact, she reacted so strongly against her mother that she actually became fearful of looking *too* attractive. "I thought that, if I looked too beautiful, I'd end up getting married and being just as repressed as my mother," she explains.

Jenny considers her mother a prime example of a woman

who fell into the beauty trap. "My mother was an actress before she got married, and she really loved it. But she thinks in absolutes. We lived in Indianapolis and she thought that, if she couldn't go to New York or Hollywood and make it big, then she might as well not try. So she got married and got a job as a bookkeeper, which she always hated."

Jenny's mother's energies went into making herself, her children, and her house look "perfect," which she deemed the correct behavior for a proper wife. Her husband appreciated her efforts, at first. "I think that my dad wanted her to look nice, but now he's frustrated because he can't talk to her. My mother simply does not have a lot of depth and my dad does. It's not that she's not basically bright. She is, but she's concentrated only on superficial things all these years."

Jenny describes herself as more like her intellectual father than like her attractive mother, in looks as well as in interests. "I've got his body type. My mother has a very good figure, although she's really too thin, I think. But I have small breasts and heavier thighs. I never did have her nice figure. Truthfully, I think my mom really *liked* the fact that I didn't look as good as she did."

Unable to compete successfully with her mother in the beauty department and fearful of being caught in a dead-end marriage, Jenny has concentrated her efforts on developing her intellectual abilities. She's now finishing her doctorate at a midwestern university and hopes to become a college professor.

At thirty-two, Jenny has never married, a fact that has disappointed her mother. "My mom has a very rigid idea of what constitutes a normal life. She's always been real frustrated with me because I don't fit into her mold." That frustration still extends to the way Jenny looks. She has opted for a very personalized appearance, often wearing brightly colored, funky clothing and very little makeup. Her blonde hair is cut in a short, pixieish style that requires no care other than washing and brushing. "I feel that looking a little different is better. I always thought that there was something demeaning about looking the same as everyone else." Margaret doesn't agree; to her, Jenny's refusal to conform has led to her daughter's single state. And she regards that as a failure.

Even today, Jenny feels caught between two desires. She'd like to be told that she looks wonderful just the way she is, a compliment that her mother never gave her. Yet Jenny remains afraid that if she ever looks marvelous, she'll find herself trapped in a marriage that, for her, would be stifling—living a life just like her mother's.

Someday, she says, she would like to be married. However, finding the right man won't be easy. She'll have to find one who appreciates her intellect and her individualism.

Many mothers see themselves in their teenage daughters, and their response to the daughter can actually be a response to a trait they dislike in themselves. Often physical appearance triggers such actions. Dr. Laura Schlessinger describes such a mother from her therapy practice: "This woman, when she was growing up, was fat and her parents didn't really pay much attention to her. It wasn't because she was an awful child or because her parents were terrible people; it was simply because they had to work a lot. But kids take everything personally."

The woman now has two daughters of her own and she's become obsessed with her looks, undergoing plastic surgery to improve her nose, her eyelids, her abdomen. Her concern with physical appearance has colored her relationship with her daughters. "One daughter is fat and the other thin. She hates the fat daughter and loves the thin one. She says that the thin daughter is everything she wishes she could be, and the fat daughter is everything she hates in herself. So she's very mean to the fat daughter."

Such a woman, Dr. Schlessinger stresses, is an extreme example. If mothers are content with themselves, that's fine.

However, if they are not, and if they notice the traits they dislike in themselves in their daughters, they are likely to attack. The daughters quite possibly will have no idea why their mothers suddenly seem so hostile.

A girl's relationship with her father, as well as with her mother, is important as she emerges into womanhood. For instance, according to psychologist Dr. Henry Biller, girls who have been deprived of normal contact with their fathers are more likely to become "boy-crazy" in their teens, as they search for male affection from a father figure.[5] Such girls may well concentrate on provocative clothing and makeup in order to attract the males who are so vital to them.

In addition, Dr. Biller feels that a young girl's reaction to males at this age may depend upon the reason *why* she has lacked her father's affection and guidance. He writes of a study of teenage girls who had lost their fathers: "Girls with divorced fathers sought out boys more and tended to be seductive toward them. . . . Such girls also tended to be sexually promiscuous. . . . The girls whose fathers had died, conversely, generally avoided boys."

He theorizes that the teenagers' reactions to men had been colored by their attitudes toward their own fathers. The daughters from broken homes were more likely to devalue and dislike their fathers. Dr. Biller feels that these girls hoped to attract a better man than Dad and that they concentrated their efforts on that goal, becoming involved with many men in an endless search for their fathers' superior. On the other hand, in those cases where the fathers had died, the daughters were more likely to remember their fathers as "idealized images of manhood, which no other man could equal."

Like the ideal mother, the ideal father will realize that his daughter is experiencing great physical and emotional changes in her teenage years. He will be aware that she often feels awkward and unattractive, and he will reassure her of her desirability while guiding her toward stable values that will last her a lifetime. I suspect that such fathers are more prevalent today than when we were young, simply because many men are now taking the time to learn how to be successful fathers. Another reason may well be that adolescent sexuality has become a more open subject than it was a couple of decades ago.

Ironically, the shame and repression that generally surrounded sexuality when we were growing up often led to a father's rejection of his daughter just as she started to mature into womanhood. It's not unusual for a father to feel some level of sexual attraction to his own daughter, just as he might to any attractive young female. However, because the incest taboo is so strong, a father may repress these sexual feelings and avoid being near his daughter so that they're less likely to recur. In extreme cases, a father may even blame the daughter for *causing* his sexual feelings toward her, although she has done nothing more than mature normally. Even if the father doesn't articulate his reasons, most daughters sense that they're being rejected because of their changing appearance.

Most daughters rejected by their fathers at this critical time suffer lifelong doubts about their attractiveness to men and about their basic worth as human beings. Because they feel that there is something wrong with them physically, they may become obsessed with their appearance—compulsively trying to fix their "defects"—in later life.

Dr. Schlessinger explains that such a reaction by a father is known as "incest anxiety," which is "a relatively common problem. The father might feel he has a Lolita growing up in his house, whether her behavior is seductive or not. Her breasts are blooming, she's having her period, she's going to be flirting with little boys. Maybe she's sitting on Daddy's lap and, like any normal person, he feels some kind of tingle or turn-on. He gets very scared of those feelings."

She stresses that such feelings are completely normal. "Feelings don't mean you have to *do* anything."

However, particularly with a father whose sexuality is repressed, or who simply doesn't understand his own urges, such feelings can be anxiety-producing. "Men push these feelings of anxiety aside," Dr. Schlessinger says. "And one way they push them aside is to stop having anything to do with their daughters."

The father who is comfortable with his sexuality, who understands it, will realize that there is nothing shameful about being somewhat attracted by his child. Unfortunately, many fathers cannot deal with the subject of sexuality at all, particularly not when it pertains to their children.

Karen, a forty-year-old commercial artist who lives in Kansas City, had such a father, whom she described as "an uptight man's man." Karen says that "my father never was Mr. Warmth around me, even when I was tiny. He would have preferred sons and, except for me, he got them. But I was the firstborn and it was another four years before my oldest brother came along." When she was a small girl, her father's attitude toward her was at least not hostile. "I didn't get much affection from him—I don't think he was capable of showing much love—but at least he came home from work every night and didn't act like he hated me."

That changed, however, when she began developing physically, about the age of eleven. "I might as well have sprouted horns and a tail instead of breasts, to judge by my father's reaction to me," Karen says. "It was as though the minute I hit puberty, I couldn't do anything to please him anymore, and I didn't know why.

"I had always been a very good student and very responsible. My father had nothing to gripe about there. But he ignored all the good things I did and spent a lot of time being on my back about the way I *looked*." Her father's comments usually centered on something sexual or provocative that he imagined in Karen's appearance. She explains, "One day, my skirt would be too short. Then my sweater would be too tight. I always wore my hair long and he said that I looked like a tramp with it hanging in my face. One day he'd say I was getting too skinny; the next that I was getting hippy. No matter what—I think I could have worn a suit of armor—there was something wrong, something sexy about it. This went on until I left home at eighteen. No matter what I did to my appearance, he made me feel as though I looked like an ugly slut.

"It took me two years of therapy to become convinced that this was really my father's problem, not mine. I grew up thinking that I was ugly, almost as though I were deformed in some way. In fact, I think I was probably a perfectly average-looking young girl. But somehow my father couldn't handle my being a girl at all."

Karen's mother was of little help to her in these family battles. "My mother was always totally under my father's influence. Usually she wouldn't say anything when he launched into one of his attacks, but once in a while, she would chime in and agree with him. She made me feel very betrayed. Sometimes I really hated her for not standing up to him and defending me." Karen adds, "You know, maybe she was also a little jealous of me. She might have been happy that he made me feel like such a loser, because it made her feel superior to me. He never attacked the way *she* looked."

After six or seven years of this kind of daily friction, it seems amazing that Karen had any ego left. "I think that you either buy what your parents are telling you and fall apart completely or you decide that *they* are the ones who are full of crap," she says. "I tended pretty much toward the second alternative. But that doesn't mean that I'm not still wearing the scars.

"Intellectually, I think I always knew that I was a fairly good-looking woman, but I still can't completely believe that emotionally. Any time a man told me that I was pretty, I would suspect his motives. Since he couldn't possibly be telling me the truth—in my heart I thought I was a real dog—he must want something from me, probably sex."

Because of her upbringing, sex was very guilt-producing for Karen. Her parents lectured her about its evils, never failing to make an example of other girls who indulged in it. "The worst thing I could possibly have done," Karen says with an ironic laugh, "would have been to get pregnant before I was married. That seems ridiculous today, when kids are drugging themselves, committing suicide, mugging old people in the streets. But in my day, with my parents, getting pregnant was *it.* And, my father left me no doubt that, if I ever got pregnant, it would be my own fault, probably because I'd lured some poor sucker into my bed by wearing long hair and sexy clothing."

Like many other women, Karen spent many of her teen and adult years firmly caught in the beauty trap. Because of her father's preoccupation with her looks, negative as it was, she felt that somehow her appearance was the most important part of her life. If she could just get it *right,* she hoped, maybe she would become worthwhile. She tried very hard to look conservative yet attractive, and she succeeded very well.

Yet, for nearly twenty-five years, Karen never *felt* good about the way she looked. Her relationships with men became tainted by her suspicion of their motives and her feelings of low self-worth. With therapy, and with a greal deal of introspection, Karen feels that she now has come to terms with her physical appearance, that she has managed to put it in some kind of realistic perspective.

After a failed marriage that produced three children, she is now dating a man she loves and with whom she feels comfortable. "For the first time, when he tells me I'm beautiful, I really *feel* beautiful," she says, and then adds with a laugh, "sometimes, at least."

Our parents, even during adolescence, influence our physical self-image greatly, but another major influence, that of our peers, takes on increased importance during this time. Conforming to our peers becomes of utmost importance during the teenage years, whether it's wearing the right brand of designer jeans or having a first date at the appropriate age.

Stanford University sociologist Sanford M. Dornbusch, Ph.D., for instance, says that youngsters start dating not when they reach a certain stage of sexual development, but when their friends start dating.[6] Those who date either earlier or later are rejected by their peer group. He cites his study for the National Health Service of adolescents between the ages of twelve and seventeen. The project correlated age, sexual development as measured by pediatricians' physical exams, parental education and income, and answers to the question, "Have you ever had a date?"

Dr. Dornbusch says that the effect of sexual development on dating, as shown by this study, is nil. The determining factor is the social activity of the teenagers' peers. "It's not in the hormones," he says. "The pressure of heterosexual relationships comes from the age groups the kids belong to. If a kid dates too early, peers reject him."

On the other hand, the teenager who doesn't date when her friends do also feels rejection, not only from the boys who fail to ask her out, but from her girlfriends as well. Since so much of adolescent attraction depends upon beauty, the dateless girl is most likely to blame her lack of suitors, and her general feeling of "not fitting in," on her appearance.

California State University, Northridge, psychology professor Patricia Keith-Spiegel, Ph.D., recalls from her own adolescence: "What you looked like on the outside was your value." When she was growing up in California in the fifties, she remembers "having to wear a uniform. When I was an adolescent, the 'in' uniform was ducktail haircuts, on both boys and girls, with a peroxided streak down the front. We looked like skunks! We cinched in our waists and wore crinolines and florescent socks. . . . I remember, even then, looking in the mirror, dressed entirely properly, and a tiny little voice in me not knowing whether to laugh or cry because the image was so *absurd*."

Dr. Keith-Spiegel, a feminist, says, "I was hoping that had changed, but I still see it in my students today. Only now it's the brand names that have to be monogrammed on your hindside."

As the mother of a boy just entering his teens, she often has an informal opportunity to observe teenage girls. "When I see girls around the house, their conversation is still almost totally appearance dominated. Sometimes I like to play devil's advocate when I can't stand it anymore. I'll say, 'Does he have a nice personality? Is he doing well in school?' They look at me like I'm an old fossil about ready to fall apart. It's only how guys *look* that's important to these girls."

Their attitude is the same when they discuss other girls. "It's all centered on the clothes," Dr. Keith-Spiegel says. "If they're talking about a girl they like, it'll be the way she dresses where they'll give her her major compliments. If they're talking about a girl they don't like, they'll criticize the way she looks. This [concept of appearance] pervades the discussions of the worth of their peers. I hear very little about sweetness, generosity, loyalty, intelligence. . . ."

This need to conform to a group is a normal part of adolescence, but Dr. Keith-Spiegel thinks that it also may play a large part in the increase in recent years of teenage depression. Just when kids are trying to find out who they are, both physically and emotionally, they are told that they should look like Brooke Shields and Matt Dillon. When they look in the mirror, they see they haven't achieved that goal, and will never achieve it. Teenagers, she says, "are so depressed. When you work with them, and ask why, they can't tell you. It's at such a level that they can't articulate what their sadness is about. Now some of that is raging hormonal battles . . . but I think these incongruities of physical perception are one cause of it."

Certainly all of us experienced the same emotional turmoil. Perhaps the current increase in depression among teens reflects not only a failure to meet certain prescribed physical standards of beauty but the addition of contemporary adolescent problems, such as the pressure to be sexually active (while most of us suffered pressure *not* to be sexually active) and the prevalence of divorced parents.

Adolescence is a time of great expectations. When expectations are not met, depression can result. Experts feel that this is one reason why young people report feeling lonelier than older people do. Psychologists Carin Rubinstein and Phillip Shaver of New York University and sociologist Letitia Anne Peplau of the University of California at Los Angeles conclude, "We think that young people are so susceptible to loneliness because they feel most sharply the discrepancy between the search for intimacy and the failure to find it. Young people are romantic and idealistic; they think it is more important to find a 'romantic or sexual partner' than older people do."[7]

Girls report feeling worse about themselves than boys do. Girls more often admit they feel lonely, sad, confused, and ashamed, according to research done by Dr. Daniel Offer, chairman of the psychiatry department of Michael Reese Hospital in Chicago, Dr. Eric Ostrov, director of forensic psychology at Michael Reese, and Dr. Kenneth I. Howard, psychology professor at Northwestern University.[8] In response to a questionnaire these researchers sent to twenty thousand teenagers, more than 40 percent of the girls admitted that *they frequently felt ugly and unattractive.*

Certainly many of these negative feelings result from a typical teenager's tendency toward self-criticism. Still, they also may be caused, or at least exacerbated, by her peers. Teens, like children, can be extremely cruel to a peer who doesn't fit their norms, for whatever reasons. That's what happened to Virginia, a young woman of West Indian background who grew up in California. While most of us had at least a realistic chance to conform when we were teens, by choosing the "right" clothes, hairstyles, makeup and such, Virginia suffered rejection because of physical qualities she couldn't change.

Virginia, now twenty-three, is tall, slender, and attractive. Her problem is her racial background, which is not clearly evident. Her parents were born in Barbados, and her ancestors include Irish, Swedish, and Africans. Although Virginia has broad features, her skin is white. And, although her hair has a kinky texture, it is medium brown. Her entire family fails to fit into easily recognizable racial categories. Virginia says, "My father is often taken for Egyptian. My mother looks more Hawaiian. My younger brother has blond hair and my older brother has dark hair. Most West Indians are from such diverse backgrounds that this is nothing unusual there."

She has learned, very painfully, in the United States, "you're either black or you're white. There's no tolerance for being in between."

Virginia's troubles started when she was young, and her family was living in a black ghetto. "The kids used to call me 'white patty,' things like that, because I wasn't dark enough. I used to get beat up at least once a month for no reason other than I was different."

Virginia's father is a businessman and, when Virginia was nine, he was able to move his family out of the ghetto. They chose a suburb that was almost completely white, and that presented other kinds of problems.

At first, Virginia had girlfriends, but their relationship changed drastically when they all reached puberty and boys became their focus of attention. "When they started to have boyfriends, all of a sudden they thought I should have one, too. We would hang out in a group of six and the other five girls all had boyfriends."

There was only one black boy, Steve, in Virginia's school. "My friends would say, 'Let's fix Virginia up with Steve.' I didn't even know him, but he was black, so he was the one I was supposed to be with. It was not fun anymore. All of a sudden, the girlhood closeness was gone and I didn't want to stay in that school."

Unlike the blacks who had beaten Virginia physically when she was a youngster, the white teenagers began to abuse her verbally. "They did a lot of name-calling. They called me 'jungle bunny,' that sort of thing. I would wear gold bangles from Barbados on my arms and they would call them slave bracelets." Virginia wanted desperately to fit in, but nothing she could do would change her appearance enough to make it possible.

Though she did try. "My hair was different—the kids would say it was real spongy, like a pillow. I would ask my mother to straighten my hair and she'd use relaxers and hot combs on it. I'd have to sit for an hour or two every time I washed my hair or went swimming, while she straightened it. And, in the summertime, I'd avoid going to swimming parties because I didn't want to tan. I wanted my skin to stay as white as possible."

At one time, Virginia even considered having cosmetic surgery to make her nose less broad, something that her mother, as well as her classmates, considered to be a "defect." "One time," Virginia says, "my nose was broken. So my mother asked the doctor, 'Well, can you fix it now that it's broken?' " But the family had a prepaid health plan that did not cover cosmetic surgery. So Virginia's nose stayed broad.

The constant pressure played havoc with Virginia's self-esteem and with her studies. Although she was a bright girl, she suffered from nearsightedness and needed eyeglasses to see the blackboard in class. With all the harassment she was enduring over her appearance, she refused to wear her glasses and risk even more. Her grades dropped.

Finally unable to take any more of her classmates' abuse, Virginia transferred to another school in her city, one which was fully integrated. "I would get up at five in the morning to take a bus into town," she says. But that didn't solve her problems, either. At the new high school, Virginia was pigeonholed with the black students. In this integrated atmosphere, the black students had no tendency to exclude Virginia because she was so light, but they shared a culture that she didn't. "I was so awkward that I didn't fit in," Virginia recalls. "The guys thought I was stuck-up because I didn't talk slang and I wasn't cool. I hadn't realized that I had lived in a white culture so long that I wouldn't fit in with the blacks. If you didn't use slang, they considered you a square."

So once again, Virginia had no dates. To some extent, this was her own idea. "Until maybe this year," she confesses, "I would not go out with any black men because of being raised in a white society. I had the same stereotypes that the white women were raised with. I thought that black men's features were not good-looking—their hair was too kinky and their noses were too broad. If a black guy tried to talk to me on the street, I'd keep going. Then I realized that I'd been a number one bigot myself. I was into looks in judging men."

The one interlude that Virginia remembers as happy during her teenage years was her junior year in high school. Her father had business in Europe at the time, and she was sent to live at an English boarding school. "In England, it was all white again, but I only had one incident of prejudice. They thought I was Iranian the whole time," Virginia explains. Overall, the European break helped her gain some perspective about herself and make progress toward resolving her identity crisis.

The return to America threw her right back into her old difficulties, however. Against her parents' wishes, she dropped out of high school. She worked for a while, trying to figure out what she could do with her life, then finally enrolled in an occupational training center where she studied word processing and got her high school diploma at the same time. Now she's in college, working toward her bachelor's degree, and finding the atmosphere there much more palatable. "At first, a few students would come up to me and actually say, 'What race are you?' but the prejudice seems to be over." Perhaps, Virginia hopes, being among better-educated people means being among people with fewer prejudices.

She dates now, both black and white men, and she wants marriage and children in the future. What color her husband is doesn't matter to her. She hopes that her traumatic experiences will help her ease the route for her own children.

While Virginia has worked hard to overcome the rejection of her peers, she still suffers its effects. "I feel very self-conscious about my looks. There never is a day that goes by that I don't think looks are real important. If one of my boyfriends looks at another girl a little too long . . . I guess [the feeling that my looks can't compete] is ingrained in me by now. I don't think I would have felt that way if people hadn't teased me so much about my nose and my hair and I'd had to stay out of the sun. . . ."

Her experiences have also caused other problems in Virginia's life. "I'm such an approval seeker, it's ridiculous. I overcompensate so that people will like me, and it's gotten me into lots of trouble." Virginia is a great procrastinator, too, a trait that stems from feeling she always has to be perfect. "I think it comes from having been criticized for my appearance all the time. I'm afraid to try. And I hate it in myself."

Virginia, of course, suffered from very severe handicaps as she tried to conform, but many of us may have felt much the same way at that age. Instead of Virginia's racial characteristics, our particular difference may have been overweight or too many freckles or being taller than the boys.

Kids can be terribly cruel to anyone who is different. I remember, for instance, an unfortunate fat girl with whom I went to school. Her last name was Larwin and many of the kids persisted in calling her Lardy. The pain that results from that kind of persecution lasts a long time and can do severe damage to our emerging sense of identity.

It's easy for any teenager to feel unattractive and, if our peers reinforce those feelings, the effects can be devastating. We will search for some way to belong, even if that search leads to self-destructive behavior. At the extremes, such self-destructive behavior can include far more serious behavior than Virginia's procrastination. Quite commonly, teens who feel so personally inadequate find themselves involved in sexual promiscuity, unwed pregnancy, or prostitution.

Cecily, for instance, speculates that her feelings of unattractiveness led her to indulge in a number of destructive sexual relationships as she desperately sought validation of her femininity. On the heels of her difficult childhood years, when her brothers constantly teased her about being ugly, Cecily entered junior high school, where she felt very unpopular.

"I was totally, one hundred percent *miserable* in junior high," recalls Cecily. "My breasts were developing and I was very self-conscious, so I walked stoop-shouldered. I had braces on my teeth and I wore glasses. I had pimples. My hair curled ferociously, no matter what I did to it. I felt horribly ugly.

"Like any kid, I wanted desperately to be popular, but I didn't have many friends. I watched to see what made other kids popular and it seemed to me that what attracted other kids to them was the way they *looked*." The right clothes, the right hair, a pretty face . . . "I tried very hard, but I never did achieve it."

When her peers started dating, Cecily was left out. Finally, when she reached sixteen, she had her first romance, with a boy she'd known since she was twelve. When she first met him, she says, "I was too ugly for him. We were just friends. I remember once I asked him to hold hands with me and he refused. I don't remember *how* he refused, but the bottom line was that he was ashamed to have people see us together."

When she was about sixteen, however, Cecily says that she "made a transformation physically"—the braces came off her teeth, she bought more becoming eyeglasses, a suntan helped clear up her skin, she found a new way to straighten her hair, and she bought "sexier" clothing. The overall effect was that she looked more appealing and suddenly the boy who considered her ugly asked her for a date. Soon they were going together.

But his early negative obsession with her looks didn't abate, even after Cecily's metamorphosis. "He would lash out at me about my body," she recalls. "He would tell me I was too flabby, I wasn't hard and firm enough, although I wasn't fat." Cecily's sexual relationship with this first lover was very rocky, but, she says, "I didn't have anybody to compare him with. He was a virgin, too." There were frequent sexual problems and Cecily's boyfriend claimed that, because of her body, he was simply turned off.

At sixteen, after years of her brothers' telling her she was ugly, Cecily was very vulnerable to her boyfriend's criticisms. Finally her clumsy lover's secret came out—he was homosexual. Because she was so inexperienced, Cecily didn't understand. She thought that, by being too ugly, she had actually made this boy turn gay.

"We broke up and I had a series of one-night stands with men for many years as a reaction. I vowed I'd never let myself get emotionally involved like that again. I was just devastated. I became very hardened and I went with a lot of different guys. These guys were real losers, but I went from one to the other."

Somewhere, she had learned to come on to men in a sexual way. Perhaps it was the seductive manipulation techniques that her father had encouraged in her when she was a tot. "I didn't mean to, but men would catch on to what I was projecting and see me just as a sex object. I wore tighter clothing, lower-cut stuff and, of course, I attracted the wrong kind of man. I didn't realize that I was causing this—I thought they were really interested in me as a person. I didn't understand that they just wanted my body."

With each of these encounters, Cecily was seeking validation that she was, despite all the evidence she felt was stacked up to the contrary, attractive, important, feminine. Each brief affair tore away more of her tattered ego. Finally, following a severe depression, Cecily went into therapy, which she found helpful.

She was able to learn to value herself. At thirty, she's happily married and training successfully for a career. "It took me years to realize that I was not really ugly. I'm like a fat person who loses weight—she's still a fat person walking around in a thin person's body. For me, no matter what I look like, my first reaction is always to think of myself as ugly."

Although the number of Cecily's sexual partners is higher than average, sexual activity among teenage girls has always been more common than many people realize. The cause is often not that the teenagers feel overwhelming sexual urges, but that indulging in sex makes them feel wanted, valued, beautiful. Sex becomes a way of getting the attention they want, at least temporarily, from boys.

Statistics show that five million of today's approximately fourteen million teenage girls are sexually active—an increase of two-thirds during the seventies.[9] The average teenager today begins sexual activity by the age of sixteen and, by age twenty, only a third of young women are still virgins. When most of us were teens, sexual activity was both less common and less accepted, particularly for girls. As we will remember, however, it still occurred, but under more secretive conditions. Often enough it resulted in pregnancy, followed by early marriage. Today, teenage pregnancy is epidemic despite improved methods of birth control. More than a million girls become pregnant each year, and early pregnancy is less likely to result in wedding bells.

According to statistics available for the eighties, of the more than a million pregnant teens each year, 38 percent will have abortions, 27 percent will be married before the baby is born, and 22 percent will choose to give birth out of wedlock. Of the unwed mothers, unlike previous generations, all but 4 percent will choose to keep their babies rather than put them up for adoption.

In earlier decades, getting pregnant was often a way to snare a husband if all else failed. And, of course, finding a husband through pregnancy was easier for the pretty girls, the ones who never lacked for boyfriends.

Leslie is a good example. Her homelife was never a happy one. Her leering stepfather was in residence until Leslie was fifteen, and money was always a problem in the family. Leslie escaped by using her beauty to gain her popularity among her peers.

"I began dating when I was fourteen," she recalls. "And I was asked out almost constantly. I wasn't very selective about the boys I dated—they had to be cute and they had to have enough money to take me to a movie or buy me a hamburger. But I didn't have a steady boyfriend for a long time, and I was never in love with anyone. I just used the boys to get out of the house."

Having many dates also gave Leslie status among her girlfriends. Although she was naturally pretty, Leslie also worked very hard on her appearance. "I always enjoyed makeup and started using it when I was fourteen. And I fussed a lot with my hair."

Clothes, however, were a problem for her. Because of the financial situation at home, Leslie couldn't afford to dress the way she wanted to, the way her classmates did. Things got worse when her mother finally summoned the courage to divorce the threatening stepfather. Leslie found a solution to her problem—shoplifting. She wanted so badly to wear clothes that conformed, that she stole.

Growing up in the South during the late fifties and early sixties, Leslie was mired in the traditional values for females. "I didn't even consider going to college. The role we were taught was to get a husband—to get married and have children. And that was it. Beauty was a valuable commodity because that got you a husband that much faster and you wouldn't have to be an old maid or go out to work."

Finding a husband became a priority for Leslie. She was a marginal student in high school. "I got straight A's until seventh grade and then, maybe because of my home problems, my grades really went down. I basically cheated my way through high school." Her priorities were dating and making herself pretty, not studying.

As she approached her eighteenth birthday, Leslie began to think more concretely about finding someone to marry. Her mother remarried and the family moved to a military town where Leslie made new friends. She wanted some stability in her life, and she thought she found it when a friend introduced her to Mike, a soldier at the local base. "He fit the description of everything I thought my husband should be. He was tall, blond, and good-looking. So I decided that he was going to be the one." In spite of her years of dating, Leslie was still a virgin.

Mike was seven years older than Leslie and much more experienced. He looked, to her immature eyes, like good husband material, so Leslie decided to end her sexual abstinence and soon became pregnant. "I got pregnant on purpose," she admits. "I really believed, deep down, that I would never get a husband any other way." Her plan worked. Eighteen years old and a senior in high school, Leslie married Mike. She not only got out of the house, she got out of high school and out of the South as well.

As might have been predicted, however, Leslie's marriage, like most teenage marriages, did not last. A few years later, she was the divorced mother of a daughter and a son and she had to find a job after all.

There are drawbacks to being pretty as a teenager, although most of us probably were not aware of them when we were that age. Perhaps the biggest one is that everything, including finding a husband, comes so easily to the pretty teen long before she's mature enough to chart her life's course. As I recall my own high school years, the best-looking girls all married shortly after graduation, if not before. Most had babies within a year. At the time, I remember envying them their popularity, although somehow I knew that I might not always feel that way.

Today, one of my closest friends, who is now a corporate executive, and I often joke about how we finally are *glad* that we weren't pretty enough to be homecoming queen in high school or attractive enough to be voted "most beautiful" in our class.

When everything is made easy because of beauty, it becomes extremely difficult to be motivated toward achievement. Why bother studying, enhancing a talent, learning to be independent, when it's so much easier to choose a husband and let him do all of those things? This is particularly true for a young woman who grows up in a society like ours, which teaches her that finding a husband to take care of her is the correct goal.

Unfortunately, by the time these pretty young brides discover that no one gets taken care of forever (besides, it would be very boring to remain a pampered, pretty child-woman forever, even if we *could* manage it), they're miles behind their less attractive and less privileged peers.

Of course, there are exceptions, pretty girls who grew up to be pretty, and successful, women. Sherry Lansing became president of Twentieth Century-Fox and later an independent movie producer. Bess Myerson became Miss America and later a New York City government administrator. Former Ford model Martha Stewart left that career to be a stockbroker and, several years after that, became one of the country's most successful caterers. But I think such women had to have even more ambition than their homelier peers in order to make it. It must have been tremendously tempting, when they were teenagers, just to sit back and bask in the attention that comes easily to beauties.

Somewhere in the middle, between the stereotypically shallow-but-beautiful high school princess and the teenager who's convinced she's an ugly freak, is undoubtedly the most comfortable place to spend one's teen years. Both extremes can have unfortunate consequences.

If unmarried pregnancy seems a sad result of the teenager's search for validation of her worth and beauty, however it is not the most disastrous consequence. That dubious award might go to prostitution. Teenage prostitution does not touch most of our lives closely, but I think that it is symbolic of the pressure we all feel—to trade our beauty for survival. As such, it deserves some inspection.

Actually, most young prostitutes don't really feel pretty. Unlike older women who turn to selling sex, young teens are often manipulated into that position by a person who seems to validate their shaky femininity. Depending upon her background, any girl with a distorted sense of physical appearance could possibly end up in prostitution.

I discussed this burgeoning problem with social psychologist Lois Lee, Ph.D., founder of Children of the Night, a Hollywood-based organization dedicated to taking child prostitutes off the streets. There are a number of factors, she says, that contribute to a girl's turning to prostitution. One, of course, may be economic desperation, particularly among runaways. Another is drugs. Among local girls who end up on Hollywood's streets, Dr. Lee says, low self-esteem and a lack of family support rank high. No one has made these adolescents feel worthwhile, so they are ripe for picking by pimps, many of whom look nothing like the pimps we see on television, Dr. Lee adds. "Many of them wear business suits and carry credit cards."

The pimps, Dr. Lee explains, "talk a good game. They say to the girl, 'Oh, baby, you're a beautiful woman, you're my lady, you're my star.' They talk circles around these kids." Dr. Lee has helped girls as young as ten years old who were working the streets of Hollywood. Other sources have told me about finding girls as young as eight prostituting themselves. Frequently, they are introduced to the life by a man who makes them feel pretty for the first time in their lives.

"Last week I saw a young girl walking down the street with a pimp," said Dr. Lee. "She was carrying her luggage and the pimp was telling her with every step how beautiful she was and how she could be his lady and a movie star. As I crossed near the child, I realized that she had a mouth deformity. She was loving the attention she was getting [from the pimp] because it was a certain kind of attention that she was not getting in her home" or anywhere else in her life. (She was the typical kind of child Children of the Night attempts to lure away from pimps and off the streets.)

When a young girl begins to work as a prostitute, her appearance changes drastically. She takes on the look of the hooker: short skirts, weird hairdos, heavy makeup. "Makeup is very important in terms of prostitution," Dr. Lee says, "because it's a way of providing a superficial kind of front."

Although to most of us the typical clothes and makeup of the street prostitute make her more bizarre-looking than beautiful, very young girls may not realize the difference. When they leave home, "these girls don't think they're attractive. Then they go on the street and they get all those strokes [from customers and pimps who comment favorably on their looks]. They get those strokes, no matter how abusive the life may be."

Street life also becomes a strange kind of beauty contest. While respectable girls in towns all over America display themselves publicly in beauty pageants, the street prostitutes do essentially the same thing. For them, the entry fee is higher and the prize sought is money. "There's so much competition [among prostitutes]. They're really on the line. What if a trick picks up a girl's friend three times and nobody picks her up at all? She feels unattractive. But the selection of a [particular] prostitute may not have anything to do with a girl's basic attractiveness. It may be that one is dressed differently or using different body language." So, quickly, the girls pick up more overtly sexual ways of dressing and behaving.

Another factor that frequently plays a part in prostitution is sexual abuse in childhood. Lois Lee estimates that approximately 80 percent of the girls she sees on the Hollywood streets were victims of sexual abuse before they left home— "if not by their fathers, then by the guy down the block."

Unfortunately, we are finding out today that such experiences are shockingly common. Incest alone has been estimated to affect several million females in the United States. A recent well-respected San Francisco study by Mills College associate professor of sociology Diana Russell documented just how common is sexual assault of young girls by family members. Professor Russell did a random survey of 930 adult women and found that one in six had suffered such an assault before the age of eighteen, and one in eight before the age of fourteen.

Walter Maksimczyk, Ph.D., clinical psychologist and administrator of the Mental Health Unit of Los Angeles County Juvenile Hall, sees many young girls who have been sexually abused and turned toward prostitution entering the correctional system. Most, he says, have been brought into prostitution by older men who initiate them into sexuality before puberty, "by the age of eleven or twelve."

He explains that such an experience, while it makes a

child feel valued in a way, is extremely harmful to her psychological development. "Adolescence is a time when girls are naturally narcissistic," he says. "Just before puberty, there is a time when they begin to primp. If she's brought into sexual relations at that time, the girl never really becomes emotionally involved in the sex act. She gets nothing from it emotionally, just money or praise. She never learns to form interpersonal relationships. These girls often turn to drugs, too, because they have no source of psychological satisfaction in relationships. They become shallow, self-caring individuals."

Dr. Maksimczyk adds that many young prostitutes are considered attractive because of only one thing, their youth. When that goes—and an aura of innocent youth doesn't last very long on the streets—they're left even more emotionally crippled.

It's unfortunately easy for any adolescent girl to become caught in the beauty trap. Perhaps the most easily learned lesson of the teens is that *beauty counts if you're a girl.* Even those of us who had ambitions beyond marriage and children knew that very well.

I remember, for instance, putting together a junior high school project on the subject of what I wanted to be when I grew up. Indulging my frequent tendency to overdo things, I wrote on not one, but *three* careers that I had dreamed about. In the fifties, a career in law or engineering or medicine or business, or even in writing, didn't occur to me. *Those* were clearly masculine fields. The three careers I chose were popular at that time. They also had glamour. And they were careers in which beauty played a significant part. My choices, in descending order of preference, were actress, model, and airline stewardess.

Ironically, I thought that by rejecting the stereotypical women's jobs—teacher, nurse, beautician, homemaker—I was being quite progressive. It's interesting that, while Jenny regarded beauty as bait for the trap of a stifling marriage like her mother's, I regarded it as a way of becoming independent of the need for a man's financial support.

Of course, I was well aware that my looks had to change quite a bit if I were to qualify for any of my chosen careers. At twelve or thirteen I was tall, skinny, and gawky and my skin had an unfortunate tendency to break out if I so much as glanced sideways at a potato chip. I felt like a mess. Yet, I figured there was still hope for me—not that I could be successful and important *without* being beautiful, but that I, too, could be gorgeous someday. I believed fervently in the tale of the ugly duckling that turned into a swan, and I read story after story about young girls who suddenly blossomed into classic beauties at fifteen or sixteen, usually knocking some handsome guy right out of his socks. Surely, I thought, it was only a matter of time until I bloomed. Never, at any time, did I believe that a woman's looks were of less than earthshaking importance.

During our adolescent years, my friends and I generally admired women who had one trait in common—beauty. There were no woman doctors or scientists or judges on our "most admired" lists. No, movie stars rated our regard, and our envy. We devoured movie magazines and memorized every detail of Debbie Reynolds's or Liz Taylor's lives. One of my girlfriends bragged that she hadn't slept for a week before Grace Kelly married her prince; she was too excited. We wanted to be exciting and glamorous, too, like Grace and Debbie and Liz. We believed that it could happen to us. All we needed, we reassured ourselves, was a way to become gorgeous.

All of us, during our teen-age years, were convinced that our ultimate worth depended upon our beauty. Our power was in our physical attractiveness.

As we raced toward the end of our trying teens, our

emerging sense of identity depended a great deal, undoubtedly far too much, not only on the way we looked, but on how we *felt* about the way we looked. As we approached young adulthood, like girls of every generation, we were already firmly caught in the beauty trap.

7

THE PINNACLE OF PRETTINESS

The ages from eighteen to about thirty are often said to be the prime of a woman's life. It's during these dozen years that she will probably become emancipated from her parents, marry, start a career, and have her first baby. Not at all incidentally, it's also during those dozen years that she is considered to be most beautiful.

When we realize that most of us will live close to eighty years, it sounds quite ridiculous to decide that our "prime" ends as we enter our fourth decade. Yet, if we believe that our power and value lie largely in our beauty—and unfortunately many of us do—we can expect our lives to peak early, before the wrinkles and sags and spreading waistlines begin to set in. Because so many women have precisely those expectations, their dozen deadline years between eighteen and thirty are often filled with a sense of urgency and panic. "If I can't make it now, while I've still got my looks," we tell ourselves at that age, "I'll never make it." "It" can refer to a variety of goals and accomplishments: being sexually attractive to men, finding the perfect husband, success in college and in a career, producing healthy and beautiful babies, achieving status and recognition in the community.

For women caught in the beauty trap, young adulthood is an anxiety-ridden time of life. Those of us who think that we're not attractive enough may try to compensate for our "failure" in a variety of ways. Yet even if we are able to compile a long list of accomplishments, we're still likely to be negative about ourselves if we don't feel particularly attractive. Those of us who are beauties and feel that our appearance is our ticket to happiness may become frantic to grasp as many of beauty's rewards as possible, before it fades.

Either route can provide us with a very traumatic journey.

Many young women today claim that they want to establish themselves in a career before they worry about finding a mate. For those of us in previous generations, the opposite was probably true. As any female who hasn't been asleep for the first eighteen years of her life has been taught, the easiest way to attract a man is to be beautiful. That may sound superficial, and it is, but there also is evidence to support that timeworn advice.

Psychologists Ellen Berscheid and Elaine Walster, for instance, sponsored a dance for college students to test the importance of physical attractiveness in dating.[1] A computer assigned each student attending the dance a blind date at random, and the students were questioned about their reactions to their dates. The psychologists reported, "The most important determinant of how much each person liked his or her date, how much he or she wanted to see the partner again, and (it was determined later) how often the men actually did ask their computer partners for subsequent dates, was simply how attractive the date was."

In another study, Berscheid and Walster compared the physical attractiveness of young women with the number of dates each reported having in the preceding year. Even though the young women they surveyed had varying personalities, degrees of intelligence, social skills, and inclinations toward dating, the researchers found that the more attractive the young woman, the more dates she had.

First dates are usually based upon first impressions. If a young man likes the way a young woman looks, he may work up his courage and ask her out. Probably not until the date itself will he have an opportunity to know her better, to determine whether or not they have anything in common that might form a basis for a continuing relationship. If he is immature, he may not realize that her attractiveness is not enough to keep a relationship alive and functioning.

Leslie had two marriages that were based largely upon her husbands' appreciating her prettiness. The first, to Mike, the military man who fathered her daughter and son and transported her out of the South, was over while Leslie was still in her early twenties. Although there had been a shortage of unmarried young women in the military town where Leslie met Mike, she's certain that "he never would have taken me out or been with me if I had not been pretty."

Basing a marriage simply on good looks and pregnancy can be difficult.

A year after she and Mike were divorced, Leslie found another husband, Paul, and again her looks were the basis for the attachment. In return, what attracted her to him was a desire to have a man take care of her and her children. Paul seemed willing. He, unlike Mike, was well-off financially. He owned several movie theaters. Because of his wealth and social status, he expected his wife to be a credit to him. To Paul, that meant Leslie had better be gorgeous.

It wasn't long before the pressure of being on constant display began to bother her. "I was a token for him to take along on his arm," she says frankly. Paul wanted Leslie to be half of a couple that people noticed and envied. He was a meticulously groomed man who adhered to the same rigid standards of appearance that he expected of Leslie. "His pants were always creased and his shoes were always shined."

However, appearances were not as important to Leslie as they were to Paul, and there were times when she simply didn't feel like spending a couple of hours doing her makeup and hair. She couldn't always spare that couple of hours either. Leslie soon had a third child, plus a house to take care of and a schedule of entertaining for her husband's business. Sometimes all she wanted to do was sit in a hot bath and soak.

Whenever her looks didn't measure up to Paul's rigid standards, he would find a way to punish her. One such incident took place at an amusement park when they were with the children. "I was wearing jeans, a T-shirt, and sandals and my hair wasn't fixed perfectly." As a result of what he regarded as her unforgivable sloppiness, Paul refused to walk with his wife, leaving Leslie trailing behind him, feeling totally rejected.

"It was extremely important to him that I look good all the time. If I didn't, he just didn't even want to be seen with me. He was extraordinarily generous with his money, and he expected me to buy clothing so that I would look presentable to his associates."

Although at first it was nice to be told that she was beautiful, and to be dressed up and shown off, Leslie soon felt hungry for more from her husband. She began to accomplish things not connected with her looks. She became good at tennis, she enrolled in several college courses and scored A's, and she wanted his praise for those achievements, too. It wasn't forthcoming. In fact, Paul found her endeavors threatening. As long as Leslie contained her power within the areas he defined as female—her beauty, her housekeeping, her parenting abilities—he was happy. As soon as she ventured into areas he considered exclusively his, trouble ensued.

As Leslie approached thirty, she became terrified. She was enmeshed in a second rocky marriage and could see herself headed for the divorce courts. The one thing that had given her any security in life, her beauty, was fading quickly in her opinion. Which was worse, to stay with Paul and be unhappy, or to be divorced and risk the possibility that, without her prettiness, she wouldn't be able to attract another man? She ultimately chose the latter course, but not before she experienced many nearly paralyzing bouts of fear.

Leslie's kind of panic is not limited to women who have never had to support themselves. Clinical psychologist J. Michael Doyle tells of one of his clients, a professional woman earning an excellent salary: "This woman is very bright and accomplished, but she's putting up with a husband who runs around with other women." Despite her business success, her husband values her mainly because she's attractive.

Why doesn't she leave him? In therapy, Dr. Doyle says, she finally discovered that, despite her business success, "her belief is that, if she loses her beauty, she's got nothing. And, because she's approaching thirty, she feels she's going to lose it pretty soon. That she can't be attractive when she's over thirty is crazy, but she feels that the only valuable things about her are her face and figure." Of course, this woman also feels that she would be nothing without a man, even if he constantly humiliates her by sleeping with other women and making sure that she learns about his infidelities.

Leslie and Dr. Doyle's client illustrate how pretty women can be victimized by marriage to men who value only their beauty. But perhaps the greater damage is done when women themselves value only beauty.

By the time we reach young adulthood, we have learned society's traditional lesson that a woman's worth is in her physical attractiveness. If we've got it, we tend to think that's all we have to offer. And if we don't, or *think* we don't, we try to compensate for what is treated as an essential failure.

There are compensations. The woman who develops her intellect and her talent, and doesn't rely solely on her appearance to get her through life surely has an advantage over a bubble-brained beauty. The sad part is that such an accomplished woman is often just as unhappy and driven as the pretty woman who is obsessed with her looks.

Eleanor Roosevelt, often described as the most admired and most accomplished of American First Ladies, is a perfect example. Mrs. Roosevelt's image was often the butt of cruel and public campaign jokes intended to harm her husband's political chances. Yet, rather than retreat in tears from public view, she excelled in many ways, as compensation for what she and others considered the "defect" of her physical appearance.

The late Helen Gahagan Douglas, in eulogizing Eleanor Roosevelt, called attention to this ever-present factor in her life: "Would Eleanor Roosevelt have had to struggle to overcome this torturous shyness if she had grown up secure in the knowledge that she was a beautiful girl? If she hadn't struggled so earnestly, would she have been so sensitive to the struggles of others? Would a beautiful Eleanor Roosevelt have escaped from the confinements of the mid-Victorian drawing room society in which she was reared? Would a beautiful Eleanor Roosevelt have wanted to escape? Would a beautiful Eleanor Roosevelt have had the same need to be, to do?"[2] Despite her many accomplishments, Mrs. Roosevelt never overcame the feeling that her lack of physical beauty made her somehow less worthwhile than women who were born possessing it. For her admirers, hers was the most lasting kind of beauty, the kind that shines from an inner worthiness—compassion, intelligence, accomplishment.

Carol Burnett is another famous personality who compensated for her lack of beauty by becoming accomplished in other ways. When she was growing up, Burnett says, her mother urged her to aim for a career in journalism "so that no matter what you look like, you can still get work."[3] That assessment from her mother stung, she admits, and she felt that, indeed, without beauty to offer, she'd better develop other abilities, in her case, intelligence and wit.

Wanda, a portly fifty-year-old Wisconsin woman who has a contagious laugh, lovely blonde hair, and a pretty face, told me that she had always been fat. As a result, "I always made up for my weight by having a good personality. I learned to joke about the tender spots before someone else did." Because she developed such a marvelous sense of humor, Wanda never had any trouble getting dates when she was a young woman. She has always had a wide circle of friends, many of whom call her for cheering up when they're feeling low. Wanda admits that she has probably benefited from having to develop more than looks. Still, she'd rather she had been born beautiful.

Joanna, a thirty-four-year-old college professor who has been overweight all her life, says, "I knew from a very young age that I would have to be smarter than other people, that I would have to study harder. I felt that, because of my size, I wouldn't be noticed unless I had something other than my looks to offer." Because of her ambition, she's done extremely well in her field. While she wouldn't give up her education and ambition, she says that she would rather be thin as well as smart and successful.

Trudi Ferguson, Ph.D., studied fifty women in their thirties who had excelled in law, medicine, the arts, and entertainment for her doctoral dissertation at the University of California, Los Angeles. She found that many of these women, earning average incomes of $100 thousand per year, had difficult childhoods. One common reason was that they had felt embarrassed about their looks. So they compensated for what they perceived as a lack of beauty by becoming successful in their chosen career fields. Because these women overcame their early problems, Dr. Ferguson says, they "seem to have learned to function in a more autonomous way outside the mainstream. As a consequence, they have been able to handle the minority status of being a success and they don't become riddled with doubt about their behavior."[4]

Many kinds of compensatory accomplishments—personality, humor, intelligence, public service, business acumen—are valuable. They can often take one much further in life than beauty.

However, many women don't compensate and decide that because they are not beautiful, they will have to compromise their ideals in order to attract a man. Such women might proceed in a variety of ways: being sexually promiscuous; providing a man with money or other material advantages; settling for a man who is less intelligent or accomplished or principled; even allowing a man to be abusive.

Regrettably, many battered women serve as examples of this attitude. Among the dozen or so I interviewed, most admitted that they felt physically ugly and, at least in part because they felt ugly, were convinced that they would never find another man if they left their abusive partner. Some of these women were not even married. Several, in fact, were not financially dependent upon their lover or spouse. Yet they were very emotionally dependent and, thus, continued the relationship, sometimes for years.

Many battered women, because they value themselves so little, are attracted to men who have a similar personality flaw. The male way of expressing low self-esteem is often to project their negative feelings onto women and batter them both verbally and physically.

Some of the women with whom I talked were quite accomplished in their own right; one was a movie company executive, another was a physical therapist, still another a civil service worker. Yet they defined themselves as inferior. One of the core ways in which they devalued themselves was in assessing their physical appearance. Interestingly, most were no less attractive than average, but they *thought* they looked far worse. And self-image is the key factor here.

Erin is a twenty-seven-year-old California nurse. Although she is an accomplished woman who put herself through college and earns her own living, her self-image was once so poor that she allowed her boyfriend to beat her, not once or twice, but over a seven-year period. When Erin was a child, her mother was often verbally abusive to her, and the insults she threw at Erin frequently centered on the child's appearance. When Erin was dressed for school, her mother would tell her that she looked like "a fat slob," and that her hair looked like "a rat's nest." Whenever Erin or her room looked less than immaculate, her mother would call her "a filthy pig." Even today, those wounds still hurt, although Erin lives three thousand miles away from her mother and refuses to see her.

As a girl, Erin fantasized that she would find a man to take her away from her unhappy home life. Her prince would arrive, and they would live happily ever after. Yet because she felt so unattractive and worthless, she couldn't really picture herself in the role of the beautiful princess. When she looked in the mirror, she saw a fat girl with a piggy face and a rat's nest on her head.

Not surprisingly, when Erin found a man, he wasn't much of a prince. Instead, he reconfirmed the negative self-image that her mother had helped her construct. Erin met Casey when she was eighteen and a freshman in college. Part of his appeal, she admits, was that he seemed excitingly dangerous, and that her mother didn't approve of him. Her mother's basic reaction to Casey was, if he were worth having, he wouldn't be interested in Erin.

"I saw him as my ticket out," Erin recalls. She felt flattered that he was attracted to her. Erin and Casey became lovers and soon she left home to live with him. They traveled west and settled in California. Shortly after they arrived, serious problems erupted. Casey didn't work. He drank too much. Eventually he began using drugs. He expected Erin to pay the bills. Casey wasn't exactly the prince-savior that Erin had imagined.

In addition, whenever Erin balked at Casey's rules, he

became abusive. It started with verbal abuse. He would call her too fat, too ugly, a slob, dirty—echoes of her mother's barbs. By now, Erin believed these things about herself. It had been only a matter of time until Casey, too, discovered her faults.

Erin also believed that men were innately superior to women. "I had all men on a pedestal," she says. She didn't want to face life without one of her own and, because she felt so ugly, she was certain that she'd never be able to attract another male. Even though Casey was turning out to be no bargain, he was better than no man at all.

Predictably, Casey's abuse escalated and he beat Erin. It started with a slap or two and, at the end, included instances when Casey threw Erin on the floor and kicked her repeatedly. Why, when she was paying the bills, did she allow him to treat her that way? "I thought I deserved it," she says simply. "He would tell me that I was too fat and too ugly, that I didn't earn enough money, and I believed him."

Occasionally, Erin would become fed up with Casey and kick him out. Yet after they lived apart for a while, her old panic would set in. Eventually, she let him move back in. Luckily, there came a time when Erin *really* had had enough. She sought help at a shelter for battered women, went into therapy, and was able to sever her relationship with Casey.

Part of her work in learning to leave Casey behind, and to avoid replacing him with another abusive man, was to elevate her self-esteem. She had to stop thinking of herself as a fat girl with a piggy face and a rat's nest on her head (a girl she had never been in any case) and begin seeing herself as an attractive, accomplished, worthwhile person.

Psychotherapist Laura Schlessinger points out that often women choose abusive men because they subconsciously think that's all they deserve. "Once a woman learns to feel better about herself, she will start being attracted to kind, caring men. She will believe that she really deserves a man who treats her well." Erin is still working on that. In the meantime, she is convinced that she's better off alone than with a man who abuses her. And that's a big step forward.

An essential element in why a woman allows a man to abuse her, of course, is her idea that she must have a man to survive, whether the kind of survival she has in mind is physical, emotional, or social. A woman alone, she believes, is nothing. Entire books have been written about why women feel this way. Here, it's sufficient to say that, because of our socialization, most of us feel at least somewhat incomplete when we are alone. Because we feel that we need a man to complete ourselves, attracting a husband or lover becomes one of the major preoccupations of young adulthood. So it's during this time of life that we may well be the most compulsive about achieving some arbitrary ideal of physical perfection in order to find a mate.

So much of this time in life is geared toward beauty. Myth has it, for instance, that all brides are beautiful. There is probably a certain truth to that. If a young woman *feels* confident and attractive on her wedding day, she probably will *look* beautiful to others. (Naturally, if she feels equally confident and attractive on any other day, she'll look beautiful then, too.) This myth is not as harmless as it might appear, because it's easy for young women to believe that marriage itself will turn them into the attractive women, the beautiful princesses, they've always yearned to be. It's another element in the fairy tale of living happily ever after.

Although young women are marrying somewhat later than they once did—as of 1979, nearly half the women in the twenty-to-twenty-four age group had never married, up from 36 percent in 1970—most American women marry during the dozen deadline years between eighteen and thirty.[5] Obviously, all of these women are not beautiful; therefore, men must be attracted by something other than mere looks.

There is no lack of opinion on the subject of what attracts a man to a woman. Marlene Dietrich, despite her famously beautiful legs, once said, "A man is more interested in a woman who is interested in him than he is in a woman with beautiful legs." Christian Dior felt that "zest is the secret of all beauty. There is no beauty that is attractive without zest."

Beauty is simply not the only quality that attracts men, no matter what we have been taught. Still, it does indeed have its importance. We can't forget Darwin and basic animal-level physical attraction.

Actress-playwright Gretchen Cryer, whose work often deals with changing male-female relationships, feels that many men react to women on two separate levels, the animal level and the intellectual level. Predictably, the two sometimes conflict. Some elements of male sexual attraction echo our animal origins, when the primitive male theoretically conquered the primitive female and took her sexually by force, Cryer thinks. Often, she says, "the more women look like 'prey' and look slightly helpless," the more sexually stimulating some men find them to be.

When she was appearing in Hollywood in the play that she coauthored with Nancy Ford, *I'm Getting My Act Together and Taking It On the Road,* Cryer often observed the young prostitutes plying their trade along Sunset Boulevard, near the theater. "They obviously have found what works with men [in terms of sexual attraction]. What works is this 'prey' kind of dressing. Very high heels, so that they can't walk with a firm and steady gait. They have to traipse along and obviously can't run away . . . tight clothing that makes them move in a certain way. It's a very calculated thing in its most exaggerated form and on a purely animal level—because nobody's out there for a relationship. They're out there only for a sexual thing."

Cryer may be right, that a man may respond physically to a woman who is overtly sexual, one whose 'beauty' is animalistically enticing to him. Yet, he's hardly going to choose a Sunset Boulevard hooker for a wife. And therein lies one of the major problems men and women face in modern times, she says. "If what the hookers are doing works, then what we are doing doesn't work. It doesn't work for me to wear boots that make me walk in a competent way. That my clothing is primarily comfortable for me doesn't work. If you wear pants or something in which you can sit with your legs spread and just be at your ease, chances are—on an animal level—that's not as sexy.

"But the problem is," Cryer asks, "how do you have a relationship that includes sensual, sexual parts" and in which the man and woman are equal? She concludes that "we're at odds with ourselves. That seems to me to be one of the biggest problems we face as men and women."

It's no wonder that women are unsure about men's desires. We receive a barrage of conflicting messages on the subject.

A recent *Glamour* magazine survey that sought to pinpoint men's likes and dislikes in women asked a male sampling, "Are a woman's looks important to you?"[6] An unsurprising 89 percent said, "Yes." Only 4 percent responded that looks didn't matter at all. Yet even with what seems like an overwhelming response in favor of beauty, we should ask ourselves just how a man interprets such a question. By answering in the affirmative, does he prefer a woman to look neat and clean? Or does she have to be certifiably gorgeous? Or a standard in between? Chances are that the relative importance of beauty varies for each man. Evidence of this might be found in the respondents' answer to another question, "What pops to mind when you think of a beautiful woman?" The largest number of respondents, a full 42 percent, answered personality first, not physical appearance. So, while beauty is indeed important to men, it is clearly not as important as other aspects.

Family sociologists Jay Schvaneveldt and Ken Cannon of Utah State University surveyed four hundred young men and women and found that neither sex felt that attractiveness was all-important in a mate.[7] More than 80 percent said that they would be willing to marry someone who was "not considered good-looking by most people," and 80 percent also declared that they would marry someone who was "good-looking but not sexy." However, more than three-quarters of the respondents said that they would not opt for a mate who was overweight.

Psychologist Joyce Brothers writes, "A poll of more than 1,000 young men revealed that personality was more important to them than beauty. Another group reported that the most appealing quality in a woman was her ability to show affection. A survey conducted by an advertising agency found that eight out of ten men want a woman who first of all will be a good mother. Seven out of ten said that their ideal woman is 'intelligent, family-oriented and self-confident.' Beauty was way down on their list of desirable qualities."[8]

Yet Dr. Brothers doesn't seem to believe her own statistics. She adds, "No matter what men say for the record, good looks are what they want most in a woman. There is quite often a difference between what people say and what they really think. When the dating desires of more than 6,000 men and women who had used a computerized dating service were analyzed, it was found that men wanted to date women who were first of all attractive, then self-confident, then good talkers."

Where does the truth lie in this morass of mixed messages? My own theory is that men may well want to date one kind of woman, but marry another. A beautiful, sexy topless dancer may make a marvelous partner for a weekend in Las Vegas, but not when it comes to bearing and rearing his kids. He might even indulge in an evening with one of those Sunset Boulevard hookers, but he certainly isn't going to bring her home to meet his mother.

The extreme of what we're talking about here is what psychologists term the madonna-prostitute complex. The man who suffers from this complex categorizes women as either madonnas, good but asexual women like his wife and his mother; or prostitutes, evil women who are very sexually stimulating. For him, no woman can be both good and sexy. Needless to say, such attitudes play havoc with the physical side of marriage, but in varying degrees of severity, they're not at all uncommon.

New York City psychiatrist Anthony Pietropinto, M.D., coauthor of *Beyond the Male Myth,* explains that the madonna-prostitute complex originates in adolescence, when the young male "suddenly notes a heightened sensitivity in his penis, erratic changes in its size, and its remarkable reactivity to almost any female in the vicinity, all of which is beyond his control. Sisters, and even his mother, are not exempted from such unwelcome sexual responses. This is more than the boy's conscious mind, already at odds with his independent organ, can bear, so he quickly divides his thoughts about women into two compartments: thoughts about mother (and similar taboo females) that are entirely nonsexual, and those about other women, which are sexual."[9]

This mental compartmentalization, however, can cause lifelong problems for a man if it persists into adulthood. Dr. Pietropinto says that "any woman who is sensitive, sentimental, caring, or maternal in any way is likely to remind him of his mother, and therefore she gets mentally relegated to the respected-but-not-coveted compartment. The only women who can remain securely in the category of potential sexual partners are those who are or can be imagined to be the opposite of a good mother—seductive, insincere, lustful, vulgar, bad—in short, prostitutes. . . . A mature man comes to realize that a sensitive, intelligent, caring woman can be desirable as a sexual partner, but the less well-adjusted man becomes sexually inhibited in the presence of a 'good' woman and, because of his guilt, avoids her or must reduce her to a 'prostitute,' as he did all sexually desirable women in his early teens."

As we all know, men mature at varying rates, just as

women do. Some may outgrow the madonna-prostitute complex before they leave their early teens and never have problems in relating to women. Many others, however, may unconsciously suffer from this complex for years longer, well into their twenties and thirties. Because of their confused desires, these young men may communicate contradictory messages about what they want from a woman. It's no wonder that the women who choose to date and marry them aren't sure just what is expected.

There are other reasons, too, why a man may not pursue the most beautiful woman available. He might fear that he couldn't hold her, that she would eventually leave him for a man who could offer her more. Or, if he's not terribly handsome himself, while he might lust after someone who looks like Christie Brinkley, he will probably feel more comfortable pursuing a woman whose level of attractiveness is similar to his own.

Following their computer dance project, Ellen Berscheid and Elaine Walster conducted several more blind date studies that showed that people of similar social desirability levels tend to pair off.[10] As a result of that later research, they concluded, "Although a person strongly prefers a date who is physically attractive, within this general tendency he or she does seek a person who is closer to his or her own attractiveness, rather than a person who is a great deal more or less attractive."

Sometimes, however, either the man or woman will possess qualities other than attractiveness that equalize a relationship with a more attractive partner. Certainly we all can recall romances and marriages between beautiful women and men who are no competition for Tom Selleck. Usually that man has intelligence, wit, career success, money, or fame to compensate for his lack of good looks. Thus, the myth of the prince and the showgirl—she may be gorgeous, but he has wealth and social status. Therefore, they are balanced (at least until she ages and loses her beauty).

Occasionally, too, the opposite combination occurs and a handsome man falls in love with a homely woman. Psychologist Alan Feingold of the City University of New York studied seventy-five physically mismatched couples and found that women paired romantically with much better looking men tended to have a better sense of humor and to "be very well adjusted."[11]

So, if during their dozen deadline years women prefer men who value them as more than a sex object, men who will stay with them to build a lifelong partnership, it's clear that women cannot depend solely on beauty. Beauty alone is not sufficient to guarantee a lasting relationship.

Physical beauty seems to be *easy.* It's passive. We women love to fantasize about the wonderful guy who will sight us across that proverbial crowded room and instantly fall in love for life. Other than standing there looking gorgeous, we won't have to *do* anything to attract him.

Even in our young adult years, we still believe in fairy tales, although by now they've been repackaged into movies and romance novels. Women from all walks of life indulge in these fantasies. For instance, six hundred women who read romance novels were surveyed by former University of Houston professor Carol Thurston.[12] She found that the typical readership of these adult fairy tales mirrors "the general population in age, education, and marital and socioeconomic status. About 40 percent of the romance readers she queried were working full time and an equal number had family incomes in excess of thirty thousand dollars a year. Nearly half had some college education.

Virtually all of them tended to believe in Prince Charming and love at first sight, the major theme of these books.

Indeed, it's a lot more work to develop other assets, the compensatory qualities such as intelligence, humor, and compassion that could provide a more ageless, lasting beauty, the kind that radiates from within. It's easier to believe rigidly that physical beauty alone is what attracts men, that physical beauty alone will result in living happily ever after.

As long as we believe in the myth that beauty is our primary value, we can kid ourselves that the next bottle of hair dye or new shade of eye shadow, something easy, will do the trick.

Beautifying ourselves physically, after all, is basically a passive activity. It requires us to take no risks, to exert little physical effort, to exercise a minimum of assertiveness or intelligence. It fits the feminine stereotype that we should sit back and wait for a man to take action on our behalf. Sometimes it even wins us a husband. What it doesn't get us is "happily ever after."

Most of us who marry in our teens and twenties choose that same time period for childbearing, quite possibly feeling that we must begin the process before we reach thirty. This choice has far more to do with physical health and our biological clocks than it does with beauty. Yet, at the same time, pregnancy and childbirth can have profound effects on our bodies and how we feel about the way they look.

In the past, it was not at all unusual for women to resent what pregnancy did to their bodies. Scarlett O'Hara's remorse over motherhood robbing her of her seventeen-inch waistline is symbolic of her era. Also, many women miscarried their unborn babies because they continued to lace their waists tightly to hide their pregnancies. In the years when pregnant women were hidden from public view, feelings of resentment over their expanding figures were certainly understandable. If a woman was pregnant, society informed her that she was not presentable. The visible evidence of her sexuality simply was not appropriate for public viewing in a sexually repressed society.

We might hope that today's women would feel differently, but some still feel quite awkward and unattractive while they are pregnant. A supportive husband who is happy about the pregnancy can be extremely helpful in shoring up his wife's self-image during this time. Many men truly believe that their wives are at their most beautiful when they are pregnant.

If they are not happy about the coming child, however, or if they are sexually repressed, husbands' attitudes can make wives feel truly ugly as their bodies expand and change. Hillary, a tall, red-haired Bostonian, gave birth to her first child when she was twenty-six. "My husband was less enthusiastic about having the baby than I was. Maybe that's why he treated me the way he did while I was pregnant." She laughs self-consciously, still trying to understand what turned out to be a major disappointment in her life. "I had had all these fantasies about being pregnant, about how we would become a marvelous, warm, and loving family. I thought that Charles would pamper me—you know, help with the housework, assist me up stairs, bring me flowers, little things."

Hillary had grown up watching all those old situation comedies on TV, the ones where the husbands treated the wives like china dolls while they were expecting. She confesses that she "probably was expecting Charles to turn into Ricky Ricardo the minute I announced I was expecting a baby. I wanted to be treated like Lucy was."

It didn't happen. Instead, Charles acted as though he were ashamed. Hillary, who had always been slim, began to feel her husband's rejection more explicitly as her figure expanded. "The first thing that happened was that my breasts enlarged—I went from a 34B to a 36D in a month! I thought that Charles would like that, but he just acted embarrassed when I asked him about it. I began to show before I was five months along. I carried the baby all in front and by the end, I looked like I had a thirty-pound watermelon stuffed under my blouse. I gained only eighteen pounds, but my arms and legs looked like sticks shooting out from my huge balloon of a middle. I had to sew my own maternity clothes because I couldn't even get into store-bought ones after my seventh month."

Toward the end of her pregnancy, Charles no longer wanted to go out in public with Hillary. "I could tell that he didn't want to be seen with me. And that really hurt. I thought I must look really grotesque if my own husband was turned off, and I began to imagine that everyone was staring at me. I had always thought that when I was pregnant I would have that glow that expectant mothers are supposed to have, that I would actually look prettier than usual. But truthfully, I felt like a cow most of the time.

"I wouldn't give up my daughter for anything, but I sure wouldn't mind adopting next time."

Not all women feel as unattractive as Hillary did during pregnancy. In fact, several women interviewed thought their looks improved while they were pregnant. That was a particularly common comment among women who had perennially fought weight problems. "I finally had a *reason* to be fat," one told me with a laugh. "I felt great wearing those maternity tops because they hid all my bulges and nobody knew that there was a fat lady under there—all they saw was a pregnant lady."

For all young mothers, however, whether they enjoy their pregnancies or not, the physical process of having children results in bodily changes, most of which are not consistent with contemporary standards of beauty. They can range from the almost unnoticeable to larger breasts, flabby abdomens, and stretch marks. Most women would not, like Scarlett O'Hara, swear off having children because of pregnancy's effects on the female figure. The joy of having a baby usually makes that a small price to pay. Yet that joy may be somewhat dampened when a mother looks in the mirror and wonders, "Is *that* the new me?"

Another important accomplishment for the dozen deadline years of life has been added in the last couple of decades. Not only do young women of recent generations want to find a husband and have a child or two before they reach thirty, they want to establish themselves in a career. The physical beauty of young adulthood can be both an asset and a drawback as a young woman pushes toward that goal.

I remember my first job after I finished college. In those

pre–Woodward and Bernstein days when journalism jobs often went begging, I landed a position as a general assignment reporter for a daily newspaper in the Midwest. My teenage awkwardness had disappeared by then, and I had learned to maneuver my five feet nine inches without tripping over my feet. I was slender but no longer as skinny as I had been in childhood. At twenty, I was an attractive young woman.

I don't really believe that my appearance was the determining factor in my landing that job; I had been a good student and had a degree in journalism to offer, along with a stack of stories I had written. But once I started work, I definitely feel that I was given special privileges because of my youthful attractiveness. The newspaper's staff of general assignment reporters included only three females—two in their forties and me. I soon began receiving attention and consideration that none of the other reporters did. At least one day a week, for instance, the assistant city editor would call me aside, mention that it was a slow news day, and suggest that I sneak out and do a little shopping. My male coworkers didn't seem to mind. Most of them were far older than I and they enjoyed engaging in good-natured teasing and flirting with me.

This routine was very pleasant for a while, but eventually I found it quite unchallenging. I was not assigned to cover murders or arson or city hall—not a sweet young thing like me! So I wrote about prize-winning heifers at the State Fair, or nurses who traveled to India to help the poor, or firemen who spent their spare time repairing broken toys so that deprived kids would have Christmas gifts. Many of these lightweight stories were downright boring. And they were not the stuff of which promotions are made. As long as I wanted to remain a general assignment reporter, I was fine, but moving up would definitely be off limits. I was not taken very seriously.

What I was experiencing at that time in my life was what Dr. Madeline Heilman's research has since illustrated: that attractiveness is an advantage in entry-level positions, but a disadvantage in higher-level jobs.[13] This experience left me feeling very frustrated, as well as unsure about myself. I felt like an ingrate to be bored. After all, everyone was treating me so *well,* how did I dare to be dissatisfied? Yet my career had stalled.

An attractive physical appearance doesn't always impede a woman's progress in business, but when a pretty woman succeeds, she's often the subject of gossip and innuendo. If she's good-looking, her critics allege, she must have gotten where she is on her back.

The case of Mary Cunningham is an excellent example. Her Harvard M.B.A. in hand, Cunningham was hired to be an executive assistant to the chairman of the Bendix Corporation when she was only twenty-seven. A year later, she was promoted to vice-president for corporate and public affairs, and three months after that, to vice-president for strategic planning. Envious Bendix employees soon began to imply that her rapid rise within the corporate ranks was due largely to a personal relationship she supposedly enjoyed with the then chief executive officer, William Agee. When the controversy grew too heated, Cunningham resigned, eventually accepting a job as vice-president for strategic planning and project development of Joseph E. Seagram & Sons, Inc. (She later left Seagrams to be president and chief operating officer of Semper, a company she formed with Agee.)

Whether or not, during her Bendix tenure, Cunningham was involved in a romance with Agee, whom she later married, is irrelevant here. What is important is that the issue probably would never have come up either at Bendix or in the press if Cunningham had been a young man of twenty-seven . . . or a homely woman of forty-five. But she was a young, attractive woman, a perfect target for the gossip-mongers.

Cunningham was angry with the way the press handled

the story of her resignation, claiming that it had engaged in "irresponsible and sexist journalism."[14] The news media, Cunningham later said, when faced with a successful young woman who is also attractive, feel "obliged to describe the color of her hair, her shape and assign an overall ten-point rating. I am still waiting to hear a detailed physical description of David Stockman, who directs the federal Office of Management and Budget and was a congressman at age thirty . . . or of Samuel Armacost, the young chief executive officer of Bank of America, who became an officer of his bank at age thirty."

When a young woman is professionally successful and also beautiful, she must be purer than Caesar's wife to avoid criticism. And that's not easy. People simply love to find reasons other than competence, whether they are valid or not, to account for a woman's success, and sex in the boardroom is a favorite choice. I'm sure that sex occasionally works, too. However, as columnist Ellen Goodman asked in her column about the Cunningham-Agee situation, "If women can sleep their way to the top, how come they aren't there?"[15]

The years between eighteen and thirty are not easy ones for us, particularly because we try to shoehorn so many major life events into them. These years seem to have become markedly more difficult in the past decade. Women who are now over forty may well have felt satisfied if they managed to marry and have a child or two during their dozen deadline years. Most of today's young women feel that they must establish themselves in a career as well. As society's emphasis on youth becomes more pronounced, the pressures on young women to perform during these years—while they still have their unspoiled beauty—increase even more.

A particularly unfortunate change, it seems to me, is that first impressions now play a larger influence on our lives than ever before. When we must rely on that first meeting, our physical appearance assumes undue importance.

There are a variety of reasons for our stronger reliance on initial impressions, most of them tied to societal changes. For example, we are now increasingly mobile. More than 56 percent of Americans do not live in the community in which they grew up.[16] That means that we can't depend on people who've known us all our lives, people who see beyond our looks, for our friendships.

Also, most of us now live in large, impersonal cities instead of in friendlier small towns and rural areas, so we meet more people on a daily basis—all of whom may judge us according to what they see.

The divorce rate in some parts of the country is now 50 percent, having nearly doubled in the last decade.[17] As a result, many of us find ourselves back in the beauty-oriented dating game trying to attract a new man.

Job changes are common in our constantly fluctuating economy, too, often forcing us into interview situations where our physical appearance is primary.

All of these societal changes increase the grip of the beauty trap on women, particularly women in the dozen deadline years of life. It's these young adults who feel most strongly that it's now or never.

We have to recognize, of course, that youth and beauty can be important advantages for a woman. Unfortunately, neither lasts.

8

FADING FLOWERS

From the time she was a teenager, there was no doubt in Alexis's mind that she had to be perfect. At all times, her hair must be perfectly coifed, her makeup flawlessly applied, her body dieted and exercised into ideal shape. When she had herself under complete control, she made sure that her children were the most adorable, her house the most immaculate, and her marriage the happiest imaginable.

However, when she entered her thirties, the facade of perfection behind which the real Alexis had been hiding began to develop cracks. Her lifelong obsession with her weight turned into a losing battle and her body would no longer conform to her youthful ideals. She noticed wrinkles on her face. She found gray hairs. Her children started to express their own ideas. Her days became too hectic to keep the house perpetually ready to receive visitors. And she discovered that, unlike the men in the romantic movies she had loved when she was a girl, her husband did not know what she was thinking unless she told him. As a result, he often didn't meet her unspoken expectations.

When she was thirty-nine, Alexis cracked. She suffered a "bad nervous breakdown" from which it took her years to recover fully.

Although she is an intelligent, accomplished woman, Alexis believes that her excessive concern with what others thought of her may well have been cemented during her teens and early twenties, when she was a frequent beauty pageant participant. "I always came in second or third, never first—except once in college." After she married, she was determined never to come in second or third again, in anything.

Alexis's need for approval centered upon her physical appearance, but spread into *appearances* in the broader sense. "I felt that I could never say, 'No,' to anyone. And every time I took something else on, I thought that I had to do it perfectly. If I didn't, I would let other people down, and then they would see that I wasn't what they had thought I was." The result of others finding out that she wasn't perfect would be that "they wouldn't accept me."

Without the approval of other people, she would not exist. She would have no identity.

Sadly, her insecurities are not unusual for women. We are taught from childhood to wait passively and attract others, particularly men. That lesson is sometimes learned far too well. We follow the fashion, not only in clothes and hairdos, but in ideas and personalities as well. Who we really are gets lost over time.

Although it takes a tremendous amount of mental energy, hiding behind a perfect facade may be feasible while a woman still has her youth. Alexis, after all, was able to conceal herself behind a pretty face and figure for thirty-nine years. Yet when the inevitable signs of aging appeared, keeping up appearances became impossible for her, as it would for anyone.

Alexis's ultimate mental breakdown was not unusual, according to marriage and family counselor Laura Schlessinger, who treats many women like Alexis in her practice. A woman's valuing herself through her beauty, Dr. Schlessinger says, "is a fuse to a bomb, because her looks are going to go and then there's often a breakdown. It's the same thing that happens to people whose whole lives are ice skating or football or anything else that is taken away from them."

A perfect example might be a woman like Marilyn Monroe, who equated her worth with her beauty. When it started to fade, she began to feel that her life was no longer worth living.

Even though there are obvious advantages to being pretty, they might turn into disadvantages as a woman ages, particularly if she has developed little other than her looks. When psychologist Ellen Berscheid compared the happiness of middle-aged women with their attractiveness twenty-five years earlier, she found that women who had been beautiful when they were young were less happy than those who had been more ordinary-looking.[1] In addition, the pretty women were less well adjusted emotionally and less satisfied with their lives than women who had always been plain.

If the years between eighteen and thirty are filled with the anxiety of *now or never* for women caught in the beauty trap, the years after thirty are filled with increasing unhappiness, depression, and self-loathing. When a woman believes that her identity depends upon her beauty, aging means that she loses portions of her identity—and her value—with each successive birthday. Some of these women compulsively visit beauty salons, try every new antiwrinkle cream or product to cover gray hair, undergo cosmetic surgery, or diet and exercise compulsively in a desperate attempt to restore their "value." Still, the day is inevitable when these artificial methods just won't work any longer.

This feeling of being worth less as we age is not limited to unaccomplished women, either. An unmarried thirty-two-year-old woman, who runs her own income tax preparation business and describes herself as a feminist, became upset after a saleswoman at a physical fitness center tried to sell her a membership by calling attention to her flabby upper arms. "She told me to lift my arm, then pinched an inch of flab on it and told me, 'Men don't *like* that!' I really had never noticed before that my arms were flabby." Later, able to smile about the situation, she admitted that "I actually went home and called up an old boyfriend and asked, 'George, did you secretly dislike my upper arms?' He just laughed. But I did feel very vulnerable, as though people were staring at my upper arms, for the next week or so—even though I knew that was crazy."

Unfortunately, not all women can find the humor in such situations. For many, the perceived loss of value inherent in aging is desperately serious. One strikingly pretty thirty-six-year-old woman has had silicone implants to enlarge her breasts and watches avidly for any other signs of physical imperfection. She is an attorney as well as a television show hostess and is as intelligent as she is beautiful. Yet, she tells her friends that when she reaches forty she will probably kill herself. She just can't face life without her youthful beauty.

We women don't concoct these negative ideas about ourselves from thin air, of course. By the time we reach thirty, we have been told over and over again that women *should* be beautiful. And beautiful for women means youthful. The more a woman can look innocent and untouched, the more she resembles a young girl, the more beautiful she is considered to be.

Our society devalues older women, and, ridiculous as it may sound, over thirty is often defined as "older" where feminine beauty is concerned. I suppose the main reason for this attitude is that women are not supposed to have any real power, except the power presumed to be in our beauty. When beauty is defined as youth, our power becomes diminished as we age. Beauty-dependent power is destined to leave us before we reach maturity, certainly long before our lives are finished.

At the same time, in a male-dominated society, an inexperienced young girl can't be much of a threat to anyone, so she is acceptable, even prized. A grown woman, however, one who has ample breasts and hips and the kind of lines in her face that come with natural aging and experience, is not naïve. She's mature and has ideas of her own. It's possible that she could challenge the existing power structure. Given her head, the older woman could be a threat, so she must be devalued. If she can be programmed to devalue herself, she becomes even less a threat.

It's clear that our society has a true double standard about aging. Older men like Paul Newman, Kirk Douglas, Burt Lancaster, and Cary Grant are still considered to be attractive and sexually appealing in their fifties, sixties, and seventies. Women their age are viewed quite differently. Jack Lemmon recently said, "People used to think I was crazy when I kept saying I can't wait to get older to play the good parts. I meant it. And it's true. The good parts really happen, for any real actor—when I say a real actor, a serious actor—when you're a little older. Maybe from your fifties on. They get richer."[2] Lemmon is undoubtedly correct, for *men* in his profession. No actress who's in touch with reality would ever make that comment. For her, good roles become harder and harder to find once she's anywhere near fifty. For example, all three television networks turned down a television movie that starred Carol Burnett and Elizabeth Taylor, both over fifty. *TV Guide,* in an article about the movie, which was ultimately produced for Home Box Office and aired in 1983, alleged that one network executive had dismissed the project, saying, "Who wants to watch an aging movie star?"[3]

According to Susan Sontag, one reason older women are discounted while older men are prized is the way in which we have traditionally defined masculine and feminine roles: " 'Masculinity' is identified with competence, autonomy, self-control—qualities which the disappearance of youth does not threaten. . . . 'Femininity' is identified with incompetence, helplessness, passivity, noncompetitiveness, being nice. Age does not improve these qualities."[4] And it does not improve beauty. Sontag adds, "Being physically attractive counts much more in a woman's life than in a man's, but beauty, identified, as it is for women, with youthfulness, does not stand up well to age."

One New York woman was so concerned about the way that older women are treated in our society that she masqueraded as one for a while to find out what her future might hold. Industrial designer Patty Moore used makeup, wigs, Ace bandages, and padded clothing to change herself from a twenty-six-year-old to a woman in her eighties.[5] Ironically, one of Moore's first forays as an old woman was to attend an Ohio gerontology conference. Among both the male and female gerontologists, people who had devoted their careers to the elderly, Moore found herself totally ignored. No one wanted to talk to her.

Several months later, dressed as a middle-class old woman, she was mugged in a New York City park. When she dressed as a "bag lady," children laughed at her and pelted her with stones. (When she appeared as a wealthy woman of the same age, however, she found that she was accorded far more respect.)

During her experiences, Moore discovered that "people either condescended or they totally dismissed me." Until she became "old," she hadn't realized just how much attention she had always received for being young and pretty.

A few years after her masquerade, Moore admitted some concern about her own aging process. "I look in the mirror and I begin to see wrinkles, and then I realize that I won't be able to wash *those* wrinkles off." Knowing what she does, this can be very frightening.

Actress Dyan Cannon had a similar experience when she played the role of Kate Blackwell in the television miniseries, "Master of the Game." As Blackwell, Cannon was aged with makeup and clothing from ages seventeen to ninety. During the filming, she observed, "I never was so aware of how people judge you by your appearance. I come out of my dressing room wearing a gray wig and matronly clothes, hunched over a cane, my face behind all these prosthetics . . . and not a head turns. I come out of my dressing room as a seventeen year old wearing a girlish outfit and wig, and all the young boys on the set give me a wolf whistle. Wait a minute! The 'me' that gets the whistles is the same inside as the little old lady nobody looks twice at. The 'me' that meets your eye isn't really me. The spirit inside is what is really me. If there's any beauty there, it has nothing to do with the number of years I've been alive."[6]

As Dyan Cannon and Patty Moore learned through artifice, and as the rest of us learn through painful experience, the years from thirty until old age are years in which we women feel increasing concern over our physical appearance, not because we feel differently, but because of the way others—particularly men—react to us.

According to New York psychotherapist Rita M. Ransohoff, Ph.D., men have very negative stereotypes of older women. Among them: that an older woman is sexually voracious; that she loses interest in nurturing and becomes domineering; that, once she has had children, she is no longer able to please her husband sexually; and that, after menopause, she is no longer worth as much as she was when she was capable of giving birth.[7] "These are images that many middle-aged women have internalized, with profound effects on their self-esteem."

An adjunct assistant professor at the New York University School of Social Work and a faculty member and supervisor at the New York School for Psychoanalytic Psychotherapy, Dr. Ransohoff wrote her doctoral dissertation on cultural attitudes toward older women. She advises that one reason men have such negative feelings toward older women is that they remind men of their own aging process and mortality. "In male fantasies," she explains, "a man never loses his power as a man and he has the power to impregnate forever." With a woman of his own age, he must acknowledge his diminishing powers.

Male thinking about older women, Dr. Ransohoff adds, suffers from a cultural lag of several centuries, a fact women must understand. "One hundred to two hundred years ago, women of forty *were* old, worn out and often died early because of childbirth. Men's fantasies have just not kept up with the new historical realities."

Before we can hope to change men's fantasies about older women, however, it seems to me that we women have to change our own. Women comprise 51 percent of American society and are, in part, responsible for the way older women are treated. As long as we consider women older than ourselves as unimportant and impotent, we are condemning ourselves to increasing self-loathing as we grow older.

Often we may not even be aware that we are prejudiced by stereotypes until we experience prejudice against older women ourselves. A forty-four-year-old teacher, for instance, mentioned that when she was in her late thirties, she "began to realize that the kinds of messages I would get from men about my looks had drastically decreased. It's really different now than it was a decade ago. I think then I was perceived as an attractive younger woman and now I'm a middle-aged woman." Like Patty Moore, she didn't realize how much attention she had received for her youth and beauty until that recognition disappeared.

Sudden awareness of getting older happens to most of us. A couple of years ago, I stopped to visit my husband's twenty-one-year-old nephew at the New York City publishing company where he works. The receptionist, a young woman dressed in mod clothes, smiled at me when I gave my name and inquired, "Are you Jim's mom?" I felt depressed all day. Did I really look old enough to have a twenty-one-year-old son? I was thirty-six at the time, and, although it was biologically possible for me to have a child that age, it was certainly unlikely.

I suppose what depressed me was the idea that the receptionist assumed I was older. Underlying my chagrin, of course, was my feeling that thirty-six was bad enough.

About a month later, I was cashing a check in a Los Angeles supermarket. I handed my driver's license identification to the young man at the cash register. He glanced at it and at me, then back at the license and declared, "You certainly don't look *that* old!" I didn't know whether to be flattered or insulted.

When I analyzed my reactions to both of these incidents I realized that emotionally I felt that being older was equivalent to being less. Why? What was wrong with thirty-six? Or forty-six? Or sixty-six? Actually, I felt better about myself with each passing year. I was becoming more mature, more experienced, more competent, more in touch with myself. So it was paradoxical that I should feel increasingly worse about my exterior.

Physical changes happen so gradually that we may be unaware of them until a stranger, or maybe a friend we haven't seen for a while, reacts to us in an unexpected way. Then we suddenly realize that how others perceive us may be quite different from how we perceive ourselves. And we have to cope with it.

This realization is hardest on those women whose identity is intimately related to their physical appearance, like Alexis. If they can't separate their innate worth from their looks, they despair. Staying mentally healthy during the aging process is a matter of learning to accept ourselves for who we are, not for who we want others to think we are. Our beauty has very little to do with who we really are.

Alexis ultimately was able to make this separation intellectually, but not until she had suffered a great deal of emotional turmoil and spent many months in therapy. Today, at forty-six, she claims she's "been healed. I'm another whole person, and I'm happier now than I've ever been in my life." Seven years after her mental breakdown, Alexis is a woman who radiates enthusiasm and self-confidence.

Ironically, part of her healing process involved consciously forcing herself into an arena where, just as in those beauty contests years ago, she was judged on her appearance. She was shopping one day in a neighborhood supermarket and "I was 'discovered.' [The store] gave me a screen test and used me in some of their ads."

As a result of this exposure, Alexis, at the age of forty, decided to try modeling in television commercials. "I'd always loved the theatre and performing. I had been in all my high school theatricals and I'd written and performed in plays when I was a kid." Alexis's father had been in show business and had offered her a choice between a college education and a Hollywood screen test when she finished high school. She chose college, where she became a beauty queen, but she never lost her love of show business. So the opportunity to try acting, late as it was, enticed her.

She made several commercials for the grocery store and managed to land a few more for other businesses. Obtaining these jobs required numerous auditions in which she had to compete with other models of her "type." She was judged by ad agencies and photographers and, most of the time, was turned down. Fortunately, such frequent rejection, based on her appearance, didn't push Alexis back over the edge. "Doing the commercials played a part in giving me a sense of identity," she explains. In addition, as part of her healing process, "I had to learn to deal with rejection, to learn to say that [being turned down for a job] didn't reflect on me. I was still a valid person. So those auditions were an exercise for me. It's not that I enjoyed them, but I did it because it gave me an opportunity to establish reality."

Each time she auditioned, was turned down, and didn't allow the experience to make her feel worse about herself,

Alexis grew stronger. Eventually she gave up acting, less, she says, because of the rejection factor than because she wanted her work to count for more than "trying to sell something I don't even believe in." So she's preparing for a new career in which she hopes to help retired people deal with their lives. Now she is much more accepting of herself. No longer does she feel that she has to look perfect to be accepted. "I had to learn to like myself, warts and all, before I got well."

Psychologist Patricia Keith-Spiegel adds that aging is additionally difficult for women because most of us are not used to rejection. "Men are much more used to dealing with rejection than women." It may well start in adolescence, when the boys ask girls for dates, risking a turndown. "That can be a very painful process, but after you go through it many times, some kind of strength builds up." These early experiences, Dr. Keith-Spiegel thinks, make it easier for men to take risks in later life. Conversely, many women are so afraid of rejection, of failure, that they don't even try. Then, when the rejection that is connected to being an older woman in our society occurs, they're not prepared to deal with it.

Alexis had to learn to deal with rejection.

Try as we might, no one escapes the aging process. These changes happen to all of us eventually. As the late Maurice Chevalier once said, "Old age isn't so bad when you consider the alternative." Neither is middle age.

As women move out of the house to become more than wives and mothers, it seems to me, we gradually are found to be "acceptable" by society for longer portions of our lives. Youth becomes less critical. *Time* magazine published an essay a few years ago that pointed to the new popularity of "older women," like Audrey Hepburn, who had played "an exquisite and sexy" romantic lead in *Robin and Marian* when she was forty-six, and Jill Clayburgh's thirty-seven-year-old divorcee in *An Unmarried Woman.*[8] The essay noted that *Harper's Bazaar's* list of the ten most beautiful women for the year

1978 were all over thirty (including Lena Horne, Candice Bergen, Diahann Carroll, Faye Dunaway, Elizabeth Taylor, et al.)

More recently, I have noticed a number of articles in magazines and newspapers on the subject of the acceptability of the older woman. It now seems to have become chic for certain actresses and models to admit, perhaps even brag about, their age. *People* magazine, in 1983, ran an article extolling the beauty of such celebrities as Jane Fonda, Faye Dunaway, Ann-Margret, Raquel Welch, and Linda Evans, all of whom are over forty, as well as Jaclyn Smith, Cher, Diana Ross, Goldie Hawn, Veronica Hamel, and Lauren Hutton, all of whom are over thirty-five.[9] Their success may well predict such acceptance in the future for the average woman over thirty or thirty-five or forty. But it's probably misleading to think that age no longer matters to most women. The fact is that the celebrities *People* cites, and who serve as a new standard of beauty for the rest of us, spend inordinate amounts of time and money trying *not to look their age.*

They have the advice and assistance of the world's top makeup artists. Stephanie Powers, forty, admits that she has to be on the set an hour earlier than her male costars because of the extra time devoted to her makeup. A movie director friend mentioned a well-known actress, only thirty-six years old, who requires a full three hours in makeup and hairstyling before she can face a camera.

In addition, near miracles can be performed with lighting and camera lenses. *People* quotes Richard L. Rawlings, cinematographer for "Dynasty," who covers his stage lights with spun-glass diffusers "to soften the light and eliminate harshness." He does this for the entire cast, but for Joan Collins and Linda Evans he does a bit more.

The effort to look younger is hardly limited to working hours. These celebrities also spend a great deal of their free time on their appearance. Linda Evans works out daily with weights in her home gymnasium and admits to touching up her hair. Jill St. John, who also tints her hair, has private sessions with an exercise-yoga instructor. Jane Fonda has built a second career on exercise. Ali MacGraw works out daily under a hot shower, to the accompaniment of audio tapes by what the magazine terms a "Los Angeles fitness guru." Virtually all of them manage, through dieting, exercise, and lucky genes, to stay a good fifteen or twenty pounds lighter than recommended on medical weight charts.

Yet, luckily, there is a growing acceptance of less privileged women over thirty in our society, and it's based on more than their physical appearance. This fact becomes evident when we consider "older" women who are admired in fields other than show business. Among those women on the list of most influential women for the 1984 *World Almanac,* for instance, are many who are over thirty. Among them are Washington Post Company board chairperson Katharine Graham; professor and politician Barbara Jordan; astronaut Sally Ride; Supreme Court Justice Sandra Day O'Connor; San Francisco mayor Dianne Feinstein; syndicated newspaper columnists Ellen Goodman and Sylvia Porter; civil rights activist Coretta Scott King; feminist and publisher of *Ms.* magazine Gloria Steinem; and tennis player Billie Jean King.

According to the *Time* essay, "Men did not initiate this interest in women who are old enough to remember Eisenhower and Stevenson. . . . Rather, a series of changes in women themselves—the way they run their lives, the way they see themselves—seems to have caused the response in men." This, I think, is the key point. We can do little to change men's attitudes unless we change our own attitudes first.

Certainly the women's movement has had a great deal of influence in this regard. I asked Betty Friedan what changes the movement had made in the way women perceive themselves. "There isn't a single image of physical beauty anymore," she replied. "There's a lot of individuality. . . . Somehow, women who before wouldn't have been considered pretty or beautiful, when they really feel good about themselves as people, look beautiful."

Certainly twenty years ago, Beverly Sills or Barbra Streisand or Diana Ross, for example, would probably not have been considered beautiful because they didn't fit into what Friedan terms the prescribed Doris Day mold. Today, I think, because these women radiate excitement and self-confidence, and because our standards of beauty have broadened, they are considered attractive as well as talented.

Still, Friedan may have credited our society with more change than has actually occurred. She says that "physical appearance has not the overwhelming importance that it used to have when women were defined in terms of the feminine mystique and were [considered to be] less than people."

Yet there are so many women who feel negative about themselves as they grow older, although many of them identify themselves as feminists. I think that it's important to study just what did happen to the active feminists of a decade ago, and their ambition of making women feel good about their natural appearance. Certainly the goal was an admirable one, but I'm not at all sure it was achieved.

Dr. Keith-Spiegel was very active in the feminist movement during the early seventies and she notes that many of the movement's participants refused to play the beauty game during those years. They wore jeans, straight hair, no makeup, and didn't shave their legs and underarms. A decade later, however, a large majority of her feminist friends have had face-lifts.

Whatever happened to their idea that natural was best? Whatever happened to the feminists' seemingly comfortable sense of self-acceptance? "Perhaps the blue jean uniform was just that—a uniform—instead of an expression of healthy individuality," Dr. Keith-Spiegel says. In addition and perhaps more significant, "they got older. The feminist movement, when we were first in it, was a *youth movement.*"

Perhaps women in their teens and twenties felt that they could afford not to conform to traditional standards of beauty. After all, an unlined face without makeup can still be considered quite beautiful, certainly much more so than an aging face. A fit, youthful body, even in jeans and a T-shirt, is considered much more attractive than one with sagging breasts.

The idea that women *should* go to a great deal of trouble to look good as they age is quite ingrained in our society, and women who fail to do so often face hostility. Gretchen Cryer found that out when her play *I'm Getting My Act Together and Taking It on the Road* opened in New York City. The play is about Heather Jones, a singer turning thirty-nine, who is putting together a new cabaret show. Heather has undergone an identity crisis and emerged determined that she will finally be herself, not a product manufactured by television, recording companies, or her manager. She plans to tell her audience that she is thirty-nine, despite her manager's warnings that admitting to that advanced age will be the kiss of death for her career. Her new material includes several songs with feminist lyrics. And she has let her looks go "natural," with her hard-earned wrinkles showing and her hair worn in her natural tight curls.

This delightful play pokes gentle fun at both men and women in our society as it illustrates the message that women are people, too, people whose lives are not over at thirty-nine. Yet one of New York's major theater critics, Walter Kerr of *The New York Times,* used his review to attack Cryer, who wrote the book and lyrics of the play and performed the role of Heather. "He said that I was trying to look unattractive, that I was flying in the face of feminine beauty, that I was trying to be obnoxious."

What Kerr said in his July 9, 1978, review was that Cryer's Heather was "burdened with a permanent frown" and "quite deliberately, looks terrible." He described her hair as "kinky-curly and . . . messy" and her wardrobe as "a dingy sweater covering a vest and skirt that seemed to have come from an attic last opened in 1914."

Yet, she says, "the whole point in the play was that this

woman had decided to let her hair be in its natural state" and to dress comfortably. "Now, obviously," she adds, Kerr "likes women who 'do' themselves, women who spend hours [on their hair and makeup]. He saw a woman's simply trying to be the way she *is* as trying to be unattractive and obnoxious toward men."

In other words, a woman who pulls herself out of the beauty trap, who refuses to squander her time and money trying futilely to turn back the clock, may be perceived not only as unattractive but as actively hostile toward men. In flexing the muscles of her independence, in demanding to be valued for qualities other than elusive beauty, she may be considered quite threatening.

The audiences for *I'm Getting My Act Together,* however, generally reacted differently from Walter Kerr, particularly the women, many of whom saw themselves in the play. "A lot of the women who came up to me after the show and who were forty-ish were so happy to hear that point of view put out," Cryer says. "Just the idea that you can accept yourself no matter what age you are. I think women yearn to be able to do that, but it's so hard in this culture. Our inner voice says to us, 'Yes, we should be able to be the way we are at whatever age we are. Our sensuality ought not to depend upon a face-lift.' But when the whole culture is geared around a teenybopper sensibility of what beauty is, that's very hard to maintain."

While there is nothing intrinsically wrong with tinting gray hair or spending a reasonable amount of time making up or exercising regularly, many women are becoming more compulsive than ever about their looks. Often they are women who have passed their thirtieth birthdays. One forty-five-year-old woman says that she began to exercise compulsively, and lost twenty pounds, as soon as she recognized the first signs of menopause. A year later, she realized that her routine was not making her feel any better about herself. "I was trying to stop the clock, and that isn't possible for anyone." So she tapered her exercise schedule to a reasonable level and began to spend her extra time in more satisfying ways.

I know a thirty-six-year-old who exercises to taped instructions for half an hour each morning and then jogs five miles. She hasn't yet discovered that she can't stop time. Her daily beauty routine, including exercising, showering, washing and styling her hair, putting on her makeup, and getting dressed, takes her close to three hours. Perhaps an actress or model whose work depends upon her looks can afford to spend that kind of time on her appearance, but no woman who is trying to gain personal independence and power in a more typical career can.

Unfortunately, for many of us, the main goal of the new physical fitness craze may be less health than beauty. One Los Angeles woman who wanted to shape up was told by a modern "fitness expert" that she shouldn't swim because "swimming was bad for me. I asked why and he told me, 'Because swimming doesn't take off inches.' " The implication, of course, is that the only reason any woman would exercise would be to flatten her stomach or trim her waist; to look younger, not to achieve physical health.

The most important reason for exercise is to maintain health. With proper exercise and a nutritious diet, we not only prolong our lives, we look better. Looking better means not only muscle tone, but a healthier appearance that results from efficient blood circulation. We need to care more about the health aspects of physical fitness, not just the beauty aspects.

It's ironic that so many of us will spend untold hours in beauty shops or exercise salons trying to look younger, but will not spend the same amount of effort improving our health. Without health, it's impossible to be beautiful. Without health, the quality of our lives becomes so reduced that the loss of beauty hardly matters.

Many of us need sound health information because during our middle years, our health becomes a concern, particularly as menopause approaches. Often our bodies begin to change in ways that confuse us, like an echo of the changes that accompany the onset of menstruation. Despite our added years, we often have no more accurate information about menopause than we did about that earlier life change.

Much of this misinformation is women's own fault, according to nurse-practitioner Ellen Nieman of the Westside Women's Clinic in Santa Monica, California. Women want to keep menopause "in the closet," says Nieman, who formed several of the first menopause support groups in the country. "They think it's a sign of age, and in Western society, no one wants to get old." She adds, however, that reluctance to be identified as a menopausal woman is understandable in a society that has so many negative stereotypes about them.

The hormonal changes of menopause can make a woman feel moody, of course, although her moods seldom shift as drastically as folklore would have us believe. Perhaps even more significant are the emotional pressures we place upon ourselves because we feel that we are aging and, therefore, losing value.

One woman recognizing early signs of her approaching menopause told me, "I spent an entire evening just sobbing. I felt as though it was all going to start now—my hormones would shut down, my bones would get brittle, my skin would get dry and wrinkled and I'd be ugly. I'd be an old woman. My poor husband tried to be understanding and romantic with me, but all I could do was cry."

Another important health concern that we face increasingly with each added year is the specter of breast cancer, which can drastically alter our concept of our bodies and our sexuality. Breast cancer strikes more than one hundred thousand women each year in the United States, and it becomes more common among women over thirty-five.

Because a diagnosis of breast cancer often means the loss of a breast, many women will not examine themselves for lumps. Some will not even call their doctors when they find a lump, until so much valuable time is wasted that they lose not a breast, but their lives. Norma Hertzog, a Costa Mesa,

California, councilwoman in her early fifties, has had breast cancer, a mastectomy, and reconstructive surgery. Following publicity about her personal ordeal, she has counseled many women who approached her for help in dealing emotionally with this dreaded disease. The most tragic cases, she says, are those women who waited too long because they were afraid that losing a breast would make them undesirable as women.

With a stronger sense of self-worth, and less emphasis on physical appearance, perhaps women won't wait to schedule a medical examination. Our value does not depend upon having two breasts to offer the world.

Ironically, because we spend so much time, effort, and money trying to preserve our beauty, we often squander our chances to gain real power and ultimately to be appreciated for something more concrete, more enduring, than our physical attractiveness.

We should take a lesson from those women whose names perennially appear on the lists of "most influential women," women like Sally Ride, Sandra Day O'Connor, Katharine Graham, Sylvia Porter. Their hard-won achievements will not fade with age, and because they have developed all aspects of themselves, they need not face aging with as much fear as other women. When she was forty-nine, for instance, Gloria Steinem was celebrating the success of her first best-selling book; at the same age, Brigitte Bardot attempted suicide because she could not face aging's erosion of her beauty. Because it was based on her accomplishments, Steinem's power was increasing while Bardot's, largely based on her looks, was declining.

Perhaps our gaining real power in the world, power based on our accomplishments, will also ultimately make us more sexually attractive in the eyes of men. That, after all, is what most women obsessed with aging are worried about. As Henry Kissinger once said, "Power is the ultimate aphrodisiac." Why not for women as well as for men? If female power is used carefully and in a way that is not emasculating, it can be attractive, not threatening, to men. We must remember that most romantic relationships exhibit a balance of power between the lovers. Traditionally, the man supplies earning power and the woman supplies her beauty, including her sexual favors. (In recent years, when the woman finds her beauty and her sexual attractiveness diminished by age, she runs a high risk of being abandoned by a husband whose own power has been enhanced over the years. In a society with a high divorce rate, the traditional power balance just doesn't work very well.)

Yet there are a variety of ways in which power can be balanced, if we are willing to consider new options. One university psychology professor points out that many men today, for a variety of reasons, are not faring as well financially as they had anticipated. As a result, a woman who offers only beauty and lifelong dependency is no longer as attractive as she once might have been. The woman who can pull her own weight economically, whatever her physical appearance, has become more desirable. The professor, who is in her thirties, uses herself as an example: "I was once an ordinary girl. Now, however, I have a Ph.D., tenure, a good income, and I've become a *prize*."

Dr. Keith-Spiegel agrees, pointing out that men have never had to depend solely upon their looks to attract a woman, except possibly during their teen-age years. When a man is in his twenties and older, women may find him attractive, but "part of what makes him attractive is that he's achieved this or that. It's not just his looks. I don't see why some day women can't fit into the same pattern."

Some already have and many financially successful women are now having to deal with the doubts that have traditionally belonged to men in the romance market. They find attractive, often younger, men approaching them and they ask themselves, "Why? Do they want me or my money?" Attorney Doris Jonas Freed, a national expert on family law, says that some of her women clients request prenuptial agreements that will help protect their money. "Some of my professional women have not been great beauties, and when they find that a gorgeous young man is eager to marry them, they do have second thoughts."[10]

It may not be until she's passed thirty, or possibly even forty, that a woman begins to realize that she must develop something more than her beauty in order to make the remainder of her life successful. Each of us is faced with a clear choice: We can feel sorry for ourselves and plunge into depression, or we can forge ahead and change.

This life crisis is among the reasons why depression among women peaks during middle age. Depression among men, on the other hand, doesn't peak until old age, after their retirement from the work force. (In recent years, of course, men have become more concerned with their aging appearance. Still, physical attractiveness remains a far less important part of the average man's identity than of the average woman's.)

Maggie Scarf, author of *Unfinished Business: Pressure Points in the Lives of Women,* says that, for many women, bodily changes due to the aging process are "a terrible narcissistic injury. The loss of her youthful looks is, in certain instances, like the loss of an important relationship. The woman is filled with a sense of emptiness and grief, as though abandoned by her beloved. It may be, however, that what she is pining for, during this complex phase of living, is none other than the youthful, sexually appealing person that she used to be."[11] The reaction to this "injury," according to Scarf, may be depression.

Some women become so depressed, and have such catastrophic expectations of aging, that they clearly participate in their own decline. For instance, Los Angeles psychologist Walter Maksimczyk says, "In my private practice, I have seen women who are so upset by their aging process, and they so expect that their husbands will leave them for a younger woman, that they literally push him out. Often he doesn't want to go—he may be happy just pursuing his business interests and not even notice that she's getting older. But her expectations are so strong that she'll begin to nag him and make him miserable to fulfill her dire predictions."

Other women use the fact of fading beauty as an excuse for a variety of failings in their lives. Some, in fact, may even exacerbate the disintegration of their physical appearance in order to have a scapegoat for their personality problems. This is similar, Dr. Keith-Spiegel says, to problems of obesity that have been studied in married women. "One of the things that women will do when they begin to feel insecure about themselves is, perhaps unconsciously but nevertheless in a goal-directed way, make themselves physically unattractive, whether it's to become grossly overweight or it's to look shabby and poorly groomed." Some studies of troubled marriages, she adds, have shown that, when the marriage starts to go bad, the wife sometimes gains a great deal of weight.

A 1983 survey of its readers by *Weight Watchers* magazine appears to support this theory.[12] The survey found that wives who considered themselves happily married were an average of twenty-four pounds overweight, while wives who considered themselves unhappily married were an average of fifty-four pounds overweight. That extra thirty pounds may serve as a scapegoat for an unhappy wife. Once she has crossed over into true obesity, she can more easily tell herself, "My husband doesn't love me anymore because I'm fat." Thus, she can avoid having to accept the responsibility for her troubles and her marriage. Her problems are more difficult to solve than overweight.

The same psychological dynamic can take place easily during the aging process. A lonely woman who notices wrinkles and sags can convince herself that people don't like her company because of her fading beauty. Then her aloneness becomes less her fault and more the fault of others. Those who ignore her, she consoles herself, have a false value system that places too much emphasis on externals. In fact, however, her problem in attracting people may have nothing to do with her looks. Or, even more likely, her problems with relationships may well have *preceded* her becoming less attractive. "It's somehow easier to say, 'Nobody likes me because I'm fat (or getting old),' than 'Nobody likes me because I haven't developed my inner resources,' " explains Dr. Keith-Spiegel.

It's also very easy not to try new options if we convince ourselves that we cannot achieve because we are too old. This has to be put into perspective, of course. Aging does place some limitations upon all of us. As a friend of mine is fond of saying, "A one-legged fat lady is not going to become a Rockette, no matter how hard she tries." True. Yet, there are numerous choices regardless of our appearance and age. But they require hard work. It's easier to say, "I'm too old," than it is to retrain for a new career. It's easier to say, "I'm too old," than it is to develop new relationships with men. It's easier to say, "I'm too old," than it is to change.

It's also a lot less rewarding.

For those of us who are willing to grit our teeth and make the kinds of changes that growing older requires of us, life can be exciting. "It can be depressing when all of a sudden you realize that you aren't going to get what you want anymore with your looks, that it just isn't going to happen. But it may give you the courage to develop in some of the areas that you've always wanted to," Dr. Keith-Spiegel says.

In her own life, Dr. Keith-Spiegel, a trim, attractive blonde in her forties, had to increase her assertiveness after she reached her late thirties. "I was always very shy as a child and in my twenties and thirties. But I was pretty, so other people would come to me. When that didn't happen anymore, I thought, 'Hey, you've got to go to them now.' "

In the beginning, she says, overcoming her shyness was frightening. "I thought that people would say, 'Go away. I don't want you. You're old.' But it was a piece of cake." Her worst fears were never realized.

As a result of being forced either to be alone or to become more assertive, Dr. Keith-Spiegel's life has changed in numerous positive ways. Any time we take control over our own lives, as being the initiator in a new relationship requires of us, we gain power. With our own power, anything is possible.

To aid us in accepting our aging process and the necessity of change, Dr. Keith-Spiegel recommends that women look for what is beneficial about growing older. Among those advantages are the following:

The declining obligations of motherhood allow us more time to do things we've always wanted to do, and time to develop ourselves in new ways. Whether we plan to go back to school, begin or advance in a career, or travel, our children's growing up and needing less of our time give us these options. I know one woman who finally found the time to teach herself how to use a surfboard when she was in her mid-sixties. There are few limits beyond those we place upon ourselves.

If we have used our years well, we become more interesting to other people. We can talk about many more substantial subjects in greater depth. As a result, we may find ourselves appreciated for our intelligence, which can be far more personally satisfying than being appreciated for our bodies.

Our life experience has taught us that we can cope well with a variety of events. Life need not be as frightening as it was when we were younger. We might take risks, try new ventures, and face the future with far more confidence in ourselves. An honest appraisal of some of our past accomplishments will help us realize this.

We reach our peak sexually in our late thirties, as inhibitions and fears of pregnancy decline. If we wish to be sexually active, we may well find that part of our lives more satisfying than ever before. Because we are more experienced and less inhibited, we can also bring more pleasure to our partners. Our romantic relationships may be fuller, too. After all, if a man becomes interested in us despite our less-than-youthful beauty, chances are good that he finds more than our body appealing. Without the pressures of youth's tendency toward instant sexual attraction, men and women have an opportunity to know each other as friends and as equals.

We are likely to have developed a sense of ourselves and our own unique style. By mid-life, we need no longer be as much of a slave to fashion as we might have been in our youth. One woman, Sadie, a California divorcee in her early forties, realized this after she attended a party given by a wealthy friend. Sadie had wanted to buy a new outfit to wear, but she couldn't find anything that appealed to her for less than three or four hundred dollars, a sum that she couldn't afford to spend. So she decided on a becoming black jumpsuit with a sheer top from her closet. "I put it on with a strand of pearls, took a couple of deep breaths, and went to the party." At first, her deepest fears were realized. Everyone wore the latest fashion, so even though she knew she looked her best, she felt out of place. "Here were women my age, women in their forties and fifties, in satin knickers and headbands. I felt like a freak." Her apprehension was premature. Soon she began to notice that "everyone was complimenting me about how well I looked. Men lined up to ask me to dance. I think that it was the way I looked, not that I was more charming or prettier than the other women. But I looked really elegant and the other women looked silly. Their outfits may have been the latest style, but knickers on a middle-aged, overweight woman are ridiculous." By following her own sense of style instead of spending more than she could afford for the latest fashions, Sadie had a wonderful evening. Maturity and a sense of herself gave her the courage to set her own style.

We have an opportunity to develop independence and self-sufficiency. These qualities can impart a great sense of self-satisfaction to us if we take the trouble to develop them. In fact, it doesn't make sense not to. The statistics are frightening; the fastest growing segment of our population is women over sixty-five. That's also the poorest segment. According to the Older Women's League, 60 percent of women over sixty-five living alone live on Social Security as their only income; four million women between forty-five and sixty-five have no health insurance; more than twelve million retirement-age women have no access to pensions; nearly three million women over sixty-five live in poverty, compared with fewer than a million men. It's clear that, for many of us, we must use our middle years to develop self-sufficiency. If we do, we will build a sense of accomplishment, self-esteem, and security far sturdier than we ever had while dependent upon someone else.

Indeed, there are many benefits to growing older and, if we dwell upon them instead of upon the negatives, we will be far happier. If we try, we can treat our years over thirty as years of opportunity. Simply in facing the crisis of aging, we will find ourselves becoming stronger, for it's only during times of change that we really grow.

The biggest problem we older women may have is our image. If we want others to admire and respect us, we first must change our self-image. We must learn to believe that we are worthwhile human beings who won't be shunted aside. Once we believe that, and begin to act upon it, others eventually will, too.

We must wrest control over our own lives. As Eleanor Roosevelt once said, "No one can make you feel inferior without your consent." We older women need to stop giving our consent. We need to start demanding respect instead. Only when we do, and when we truly believe we deserve it, will we look and feel beautiful—at any age.

9

THE FAT FIXATION

Americans now spend $14 billion a year on diets and diet products.[1] A Virginia Slims American Women's Opinion Poll found that one out of six women is on a diet *all the time.*[2] According to a *Glamour* magazine survey, almost half of American women are on a diet *most* of the time and a full half feel guilty if they overeat.[3] Seventy-eight percent of the women questioned by *Glamour* think they are naturally overweight.

Yet, despite all this concern about weight and all this effort to lose extra pounds, a significant portion of American women are at last 20 percent overweight: 25 percent of the thirty to thirty-nine age group; 40 percent of the forty to forty-nine age group; and 46 percent of the fifty to fifty-nine age group.[4]

In short, many women are literally obsessed with their figures and their weight. Some may achieve the thin body of their ideal, but because today's standard is abnormally slender, very few accomplish this without great effort. Most women who reduce to model thinness rely on strict self-denial, frenetic exercising, health-threatening diet plans and pills, or bizarre eating habits. Those women who fall short of their goals, even though they may be within weight-chart health standards, often feel guilty and ashamed about their "failures." For many of us living in today's diet-conscious culture, being fat has become the equivalent of being not only ugly, but sinful as well.

There's ample evidence that the ideal female shape has indeed become thinner in recent years. Marilyn Monroe would be considered chubby by today's standards, yet in her day she was the epitome of voluptuous femininity. Today's pared-down standard might be Victoria Principal or Brooke Shields.

One group of researchers documented this trend toward slenderness by examining data from Miss America Pageants and *Playboy* centerfolds over a twenty-year period.[5] During this same period, there was also a significant increase in the number of diet articles appearing in six women's magazines that they surveyed, according to David M. Garner and Paul E. Garfinkel of Clarke Institute of Psychiatry and Donald Schwartz and Michael Thompson of Michael Reese Hospital and Medical Center.

Ironically, however, these researchers found that, while our "ideal beauty" has become slimmer, the rest of us have actually put on a few pounds. The gap between our own body shapes and those of our role models has widened and, as a result, many of us disapprove of the body we see in the mirror. Predictably, our dissatisfaction with our bodies quickly becomes dissatisfaction with ourselves.

In their research report, Garner, Garfinkel, Schwartz, and Thompson also cite other medical and psychological researchers who have connected weight with self-image in women. One such study showed that self-satisfaction decreased as personal body size deviated from the social stereotype. Another found that as many as 70 percent of high school girls were unhappy enough with their appearance to try to lose weight. A number of researchers and writers have linked today's social pressure to be thin to increases in the incidence of anorexia nervosa, bulimia, and related eating disorders. At an extreme, they report, thinness is even related to a cessation of the menstrual cycle. Thus, "it is ironic that the current symbol of 'sexual attractiveness' may be gravitating toward a weight which is in . . . opposition to normal reproductive activity."

During times of famine and hardship, body fat becomes a symbol of wealth and status, but the opposite is true in today's relatively affluent times. As the old saying states, "You can never be too rich or too thin." And rich and thin are definitely connected. Social class is a powerful determinant of obesity, according to Albert Stunkard, M.D., professor of psychiatry at the University of Pennsylvania. Dr. Stunkard's research in New York City compared that city's wealthy women with those living on the working class Lower East Side. "The lower classes tended to be far more obese than the upper classes, but this is much more prevalent in women than in men. We found six times as much correlation between social class and obesity in women as in men." Two reasons for this discrepancy, Dr. Stunkard says, may be that women are more exposed to food than men are and that the upper classes value thinness in women more than in men.

According to prevailing values, those wealthy enough to eat anything and everything they desire must exhibit their superior self-control through remaining slender. Because self-image and identity are far more closely tied to a woman's physical appearance than to a man's, wealthy women feel more pressure to conform to these standards than do their husbands and fathers.

"It's what they call eco-chic," says Dr. Margaret Mackenzie, anthropologist and research fellow at the University of California, Berkeley, who has spent several years studying what she calls "the national obsession about obesity."[6] According to Dr. Mackenzie, "in a nation that's brimming over with junk food, being really thin demonstrates that you have self-control. You are in control of your life, and that appears to be the ambition of many Americans today." She notes that many Europeans, too, are beginning to follow the American lead in weight control.

The mass media, of course, constantly reinforce the cult of slenderness for us. Each time we turn on the television set, go to the movies, or open a fashion magazine, we see beautiful thin women presented favorably. If heavy women are photographed, they're shown as life's losers.

In our culture, thinness has become a symbol of self-control, of social status, of worthiness, of femininity. As a result, those of us who are not thin or (heaven forbid!) are actually fat are deemed just the opposite—lacking in self-control, low in social status, unworthy, unfeminine. Society treats us unkindly, often from childhood. Eventually, we internalize these negative messages and learn to feel inferior, all because our bodies are not perfect.

Fifty-year-old Wanda, who still has a flawless ivory complexion and soft ash blonde hair, has battled a weight problem all her life. Growing up in a small Wisconsin town as the only daughter of a widowed mother, Wanda remembers the pain of being fat. "When I was a child, I can remember my mother telling me that I was going to be heavy—both of my grandmothers weighed over two hundred pounds." Despite her probable genetic predisposition to overweight, Wanda was taught in a variety of ways that fat was bad. "My mother was always putting me on diets. I would not be allowed to put sugar on my cereal, for example. But she fed me peanut butter. The diets didn't work."

Wanda learned early in life that other children can be very cruel. "I was enough overweight as a child that the other kids were prejudiced against me. I wasn't included on teams because I couldn't run well enough. . . ." Also, her clothes set her apart. "As a child, I had to wear the chubbiettes sizes. They were terrible—puffed sleeves and ties in the back." Wanda regarded the clothes as another way in which she was made to look different from her peers.

When she was still quite young, Wanda realized that she had a choice: she could withdraw and feel sorry for herself, or she could find some way to compensate for her extra pounds. She chose the latter. Wanda's mother had taught her that, because she was heavy, other people would assume that she was also dirty; therefore, she must always be extra clean about herself and her home. Wanda followed that advice for years. She also compensated in another way, developing a personality and sense of humor that have held her in good stead all these years. But her efforts exacted a price. She became fanatic about cleanliness, and although "I had a good personality," she says frankly, "inside I felt awful about myself."

Her mother's remarriage when Wanda was eight didn't alleviate those feelings of inadequacy. She acquired several stepsiblings, one of whom was a girl her own age. "I think it was my stepsister who had a big influence on me. She was thin and she was always saying that if you were overweight and uneducated, you were nothing. I didn't go past high school and I was always fat, so I felt I was nothing."

Wounds we receive in our youth heal slowly; sometimes they never heal at all. During her high school years, Wanda decided that she was not going to limit herself just because she was fat. She became a cheerleader and a drum majorette. "In high school, my weight didn't hinder me so much physically." She adds with the self-deprecatory laugh that is her trademark, "When you come from a town of three hundred people, you can jump high enough to qualify even if you *do* weigh 165."

Wanda had advantages over many of the other overweight girls in her class. She was not as fat as some. ("There were a few who weighed over two hundred") and she has a pretty face and lovely hair. At five feet two, she was able to avoid looking as immense as some of the girls who were both tall and heavy. Wanda was able to keep the pain she felt, for herself and the other fat girls as well, buried beneath her mirthful exterior. "Sometimes the kids would be cruel to the other girls who were overweight and I would feel their hurt. When we had a carnival one time, someone said that we should make Florence the float—she was one of the fattest girls. I really felt bad for her.

"And I also remember one time a boy referred to me in the school newspaper as a fatso. That hurt like crazy, but I wouldn't let anyone know that. I laughed harder than anybody else."

Despite her weight, Wanda managed to achieve popularity in high school. She dated several boys, none of whom ever commented about her weight. Still, she felt self-conscious about dating, largely because she thought she didn't wear clothes well. "I didn't want to wear bathing suits or sundresses and my boots wouldn't zip. It's harder to be attractive when you're heavy. I wanted to be more like everybody else, but I wasn't willing to give up malts and chocolate cake." Even so, Wanda was married two days after her high school graduation. "I got down to 145 pounds for my wedding, but I gained back twenty pounds on my honeymoon."

Being married didn't help Wanda's flagging self-image. Her husband, Sam, was a thin man. "Believe me, when you weigh more than your husband, it's hard to take." Sam never criticized her for being fat, but his family managed to make snide remarks within Wanda's hearing. "They would never say anything about me specifically, just about fat people in general. My sister-in-law in particular made me feel bad. For example, she might say that when old Aunt Louise stands sideways, you can't see her kitchen sink."

Her mother's old messages were well learned. "My mother had nail polish on her fingernails when she died. I can still remember that. She was always going at herself with a file or tweezers and a magnifying mirror and I became the same way." Wanda became even more compulsive about keeping herself and her house spotless. "I can joke about it now," she confesses, "but I practically boiled my own nipples when I was going to nurse one of my babies." There were plenty of babies. Wanda had five children in eleven years. "I was careful about their diets when they were little," Wanda says, but admits that "part of that was that I didn't want them to make a mess. I had a high chair that was red with chrome all over it. I wouldn't butter the kids' bread because it would get the chrome all messy." Luckily, in Wanda's opinion, all of her children inherited Sam's body type and have managed to avoid what she considers to be the curse of overweight.

It wasn't until she was nearly forty that Wanda began to question her compulsive cleanliness. "The turning point in my life was one day when a tornado came through town." None of her family was hurt and their house wasn't touched, but Wanda was deeply affected by the destruction. "Prior to that, I'd been a perfect housekeeper, but suddenly I realized that everything can be wiped out in seconds." She reconsidered her value system and decided that "*Better Homes and Gardens* would never come to take pictures—at least not of *my* house." She decided to change her priorities, stop hiding in her spotless home, and find a job.

Today, Wanda is married to her second husband. She and Sam were divorced after she went to work, which changed her life-style. He preferred her fat and housebound. Her children are grown and on their own.

Wanda still keeps a neat house, but is not afraid to allow a visitor to see it in a less-than-perfect state. Cleanliness is no longer an antidote for obesity. Over the years, she's developed a much improved sense of self-acceptance; but it's not total yet. Every once in a while she is shocked to discover that it still hurts her when someone makes a cruel or thoughtless remark about overweight people. "Last week I went into [a clothing store for larger women]. There were these two women walking by as I came out—they didn't look so wonderful themselves, by the way. One said to the other, 'Oh, that's where all the old fat ladies shop.' I heard her and it really got to me. I came home almost in tears.

"But the hardest thing was that I thought I had gotten over caring about all that stuff. Those old tapes just started playing in my head again. Here I am, fifty years old, going on fifty-one, and I still feel hurt."

Wanda, like most heavy women, has tried her share of diets over the years. The weight always returns. Even when she was thinner, she didn't consider herself thinner. Looking in the mirror, she still saw a fat woman standing there, even though friends commented favorably on her weight loss.

Wanda's experience is a common one for women who have long been heavy and suddenly lose weight. Baila Zeitz, Ph.D., a New York City psychologist, says, "One of the big problems women may have with a major weight loss is that they don't absorb the fact that they look very different. They still see themselves as fat, and they are astonished when they get feedback. Suddenly they get a lot of sexual attention; this experience can be freaky and, for some, negative."[7]

For others, however, finally getting attention from men can be a heady experience. Susan felt that way while she was in graduate school. She dieted her five-feet-six-inch frame down to 125 pounds and "was very thin. I was actually a normal-sized person at that time."

Finally men noticed her in a positive way. As a little girl, her father had thought she was pretty, but often urged her to lose weight. Her brother had delighted in taunting her by calling her "pachyderm." She dated occasionally in high school and college, but her dates "never seemed to be the best-looking fellows or the ones I wanted the most. *They* were off with the good-looking girls." In graduate school, many pounds lighter and a thousand miles away from home, Susan finally experienced the popularity with men that she had dreamed about so often. "I dated more in my year in graduate school than in the previous five years combined.

"I hit that campus and there were guys all over the place wanting to date me." She changed the way she dressed. "I became much more interested in the clothes I wore. I wore makeup. I wore bright colors. I never would have picked those clothes two years earlier." Growing up, Susan's wardrobe consisted largely of one color—solid black. "My mother's point of view was that black makes you look thinner," she explains.

"I even became conscious of the way I sat. I remember one Saturday morning I was working in the campus library. I was sitting at the desk with my hair falling over my face in a certain way and this guy I was dating commented that I looked beautiful with my hair like that. I told him, 'I know. I'm sitting like that on purpose.'

"I was aware of what I was doing, but I couldn't quite pull off pretending it was natural. [My frankness] struck him as very funny and he said, 'You're not supposed to tell me things like that.' But this [game] was all very new to me."

Susan, now thirty-six and still battling her tendency toward overweight, enjoyed the sexual attention. In fact, she met her husband in graduate school. Yet not all women feel comfortable attracting men, and they may gain weight in order to avoid having to deal with them or with sex.

That happened to formerly thin Leslie following her second divorce. "I gained about thirty-five pounds and I've been struggling with my weight ever since. Every time I've dieted and gotten thin, another man comes into my life and brings problems to me, so my weight goes right back up again." In therapy, Leslie learned that she is "protecting myself with layers of fat, to keep myself away from men. Probably I fear men deep down anyway. I fear the feelings of helplessness and dependency that I've developed toward them." She also fears their rejection, as well as having to reject them. Relationships "never turn out the way I want them to," she says wistfully, so she's found a simple way to protect herself from having to deal with them—her extra weight.

Most experts would agree with Leslie's therapist that obesity has a psychological base, as do anorexia and bulimia.

Food carries various symbolic meanings for all of us, a common one being comfort. When we were children, food was very likely an important treat. "Be a good girl and I'll give you a cookie," Mom probably offered more than once. So it became a reward. Or, "Dry your tears and have an ice-cream cone." Thus, food became symbolic of nurturance. Consequently, when we feel blue in later years, we may eat to comfort ourselves. Unfortunately, when we eat we gain more weight, which in turn makes us less attractive. When we're less attractive, we become even less likely to receive nonfattening nurturance from other people. We become caught in another vicious circle.

According to London doctors Peter Daily and Joan Gomez, who specialize in eating disorders, "In the long run, all obesity is psychological." They believe that the obese person often uses food as a tranquilizer, and it is such an effective one that as she becomes fatter, she actually no longer feels emotions like anxiety or depression. The emotions of the obese person are neutered with food. In fact, the doctors claim, unless the obese reduce to within about 25 percent above their normal weight, they cannot even consciously grasp that they have any psychological problems. (In the case of anorexics, they must gain to within 84 percent of their normal weight.) In other words, psychological therapy can't help either overeaters or undereaters until their weight is stabilized near normal limits.

Dr. Albert Stunkard says that behavior therapy programs are often the most effective way to help compulsive eaters lose weight. "We try to teach people to control their own lives, not to be controlled by their environment. Try to find out what you're really doing—each time you eat, write down what you ate, what time it was, what you were feeling, who you were with at the time, how hungry you felt, maybe even how many calories you ate. You will begin to see a pattern, probably showing that you're not eating in response to hunger, but in response to something else."

Among the reasons people overeat, Dr. Stunkard says, is to help them handle such unpleasant emotions as boredom, anger, frustration, and anxiety. He advises us to learn to recognize what we're doing when we eat unnecessarily, then to work out a strategy for dealing with the situation in a more useful way. "The strategy may not even work, but you'll feel better for having tried." Such overt efforts will help raise the heavy person's self-esteem, which is an essential ingredient for losing weight and keeping it off. "If you don't have self-esteem, you will be able to do nothing to alleviate your situation, your feelings of frustration and helplessness [will get worse] and you'll eat more."

Losing weight, for the chronically obese person, is far from an easy task. Because of society's pressures, on women in particular, to be slender, few fat women enjoy self-esteem. With great effort and behavior modification, however, overweight women do manage to slim down. Then they may face more, if different, problems, such as negative reactions from family and friends. "I lost fifty pounds once," Wanda recalls, "but my husband shot me down. I got a lot of compliments on the way I looked, but he kept saying that he couldn't see the difference at all. I think he didn't want me to lose weight. We would go out more often and he would push me to go to restaurants, to fatten me up again."

Why this may happen is not difficult to understand. When we make any major alteration in our lives, we risk threatening those closest to us. With change, the balance of power in a relationship shifts and that can create discomfort, particularly for the person who has not changed. Dr. Charles Lucas, clinical nutrition unit director of Detroit's Wayne State University Health Center, says it's common for spouses to torpedo their partners' diets, offering them forbidden foods and cooking their favorite dishes.[8] Losing weight exhibits control and "a lot of people are envious of other people who take charge of their lives. They wonder what's going to come next, and whether the relationship is going to change."

An attractive woman in her thirties admits that, when she was sixty pounds overweight, her husband constantly criticized her ample figure. Yet when she began dieting seriously and slimming down from obese to normal, he brought her boxes of her favorite candies. For him, the misery of the past was more comfortable than an uncertain future. When his wife lost weight, he responded to her as an attractive woman once again. So might other men. A thin wife might leave him for someone else.

Again the key issue is self-esteem. It's hard for a heavy woman to feel good about herself in our society, though some do manage. The magazine *Big Beautiful Woman* is dedicated to elevating the image of the overweight female. Several designers are creating very attractive clothing for the size sixteen-plus figure.

One woman who has managed career success and a healthy dose of good feelings about herself despite a size eighteen physique is Phyllis Eliasberg, consumer reporter for WABC-TV in New York City. Eliasberg, who is in her forties, dresses mainly in smocks in a variety of solid colors and prints. Her blonde hair is perfectly coifed and her makeup expertly applied as she does her daily stint on the five o'clock news.

Eliasberg is a highly accomplished and intelligent woman who has managed to feel good about herself despite a weight problem that got worse "when I quit smoking ten years ago." At that time she was an attorney in Los Angeles. She was invited to use her legal knowledge as consumer reporter for KNXT-TV in Los Angeles and, before long, was smitten with the idea of appearing before an audience.

"When I started in television," she says with her ever-present sense of humor, "I was a gorgeous size ten, with this mane of blonde hair—really dynamite. That was for fifteen minutes of my life."

Over the following years, Eliasberg moved from Los Angeles to WXYZ-TV in Detroit, and finally to WABC-TV. But, as she added years of experience to her resume, she added pounds to her figure as well. When she hit New York City a couple of years ago, she was definitely overweight, and *then* she discovered the Big Apple's restaurants.

Eliasberg thinks that she may be "the only fat female TV reporter in the country." A woman her size, in her appearance-conscious profession, she admits, is "unusual. I have never seen another fat woman reporter. But I've seen fat men. Charles Kuralt. No one questions him—'Charlie, has your fat stood in your way?' " She laughs. "And Andy Rooney. Andy Rooney is, indeed, portly." The double standard reigns in television as in most of life. "I'm the only reporter in TV who can have a charge account at Lane Bryant."

Because she's one of the few large women on television, Eliasberg has become something of a role model for other heavy women. "I spoke at a women's luncheon in Scarsdale, and a woman came up to me and said, 'I am so glad that you are not a size three. It is such a comfort to know that somebody of our proportions can make it.' And, you know, I do shop at Lane Bryant and a lot of the women I meet there are really pleased that I'm on television."

She realizes that not everyone is supportive, however. "I'm sure that there are people who look at me and think, 'That fat thing. Why doesn't she get control and go on a diet?' I'm certain that happens. And I've had women [viewers] call me up and say, '*We* really should go on a diet,' because they've got the problem, too."

Eliasberg doesn't let such negative attitudes get her down. "You know, I tell them, 'I really have to accept myself the way I am and, at the moment, I'm fat. It's okay that I'm not a size twelve.' I really have to do that, or I couldn't function. I am, sort of, content.

"I would love to be a size twelve, if it were magic, but I'm not willing to make the effort systematically."

Self-acceptance, Phyllis Eliasberg has learned, is what every woman needs. She's been able to achieve it, at least most of the time. "I am not gorgeous," she says frankly. "I am not slim. I am not young. I have grown children and I'm middle-aged. Nevertheless, my life is an adventure. It really is such a wonderful adventure.

"I can't stop and worry about the fat."

Yet most of us do just that. Because we buy the idea that thin is best, we squander our emotions, our time, our money, even our physical and mental health in trying to achieve a thin body.

For most of us, the health risks of overweight may well be less than those of constant dieting. Many doctors believe that the health problems of overweight, such as high blood pressure, heart attack, stroke, and diabetes, become significant only when a person weighs at least 35 percent more than the optimum weight. For my height of five feet nine inches, my medium frame would have to weigh more than 200 pounds before I would be considered medically obese.[9] I've never come anywhere close to weighing that much, but I've certainly looked in the mirror more than once and hated my image, cataloging every bulge, real or imagined, as though it were concrete evidence of my shortcomings. The woman of average height, five feet four inches, would have to weigh more than 180 before reaching obese standards.

Most American women are not obese. For those who are, there are very real health risks. Most of us, however, are battling only ten or twenty extra pounds. Ironically, statistics show that people who are no more than twenty pounds overweight often live longer than those who stay thin. (Dr. Reubin Andres of the National Institute on Aging suspects the reason for this phenomenon may be that a little surplus weight serves as a "reserve" that helps slightly overweight people survive illnesses.[10]) For most of us, the reasons why we want to weigh less are not medical. They're purely cosmetic, and our constant dieting may well be harming our health far more than a few extra pounds could.

One woman, a slender blonde in her mid-twenties, told me that her husband had removed the bathroom scale from their home because he could no longer take her moodiness. "I would get up in the morning and weigh myself. And then I'd weigh myself after each meal. If I gained a fraction of an ounce anywhere along the line, my day would be shot."

A friend of mine who just turned forty and who perpetually weighs perhaps ten pounds more than she'd like to finally cured her own obsession with the scale by refusing to look at one. The only time she is weighed is when she goes for her annual physical exam, and then she stands with her back to the scale's balance beam, instructing the doctor not to tell her what she weighs. "It may sound crazy," she explains, "but I think I'm better off not knowing. If my clothes start getting tight, I cut back on what I eat. And I exercise, because I know it's good for me. But if I have real numbers to worry about, I become absolutely compulsive about losing weight. The only way I can stop is not to know how much I weigh."

Probably any woman who's ever tried to diet can understand how these women feel. Dr. Margaret Mackenzie points out that "concentrating on a diet actually increases the obsession with the problem we are trying to eliminate."

There were years in which I would diet, too, but I finally gave it up. Each time I tried to lose weight, I would actually gain instead. Thinking about *food* all the time just made me hungry, and next thing I knew, I was cheating like mad. I was caught most firmly in the beauty trap when I was on a diet. I felt depressed and ugly. So I ate.

When I was able to forget about my weight, and instead concentrate on eating healthy foods and exercising for half an hour several days a week, I ended up weighing less than I did when I dieted. Actually, there's scientific evidence that I might have had similar results even if I hadn't cheated on my diets. A study of one hundred teenage Canadian girls bears this out. Those with poor and restricted eating habits weighed more than those with nutritionally sound diets, although the heavier girls ate an average of only twelve hundred calories a day while the slimmer ones ate an average of twenty-three hundred calories.[11] One of the study's coauthors, Lorry A. Macdonald of McMaster University in Hamilton, Ontario, says that appearance becomes a major influence on eating habits. Macdonald concludes that "it's a vicious cycle. The heavier girls were trying to improve their looks, but because their calorie intake was low, they didn't have the energy for any kind of activity. The girls who were happy with their appearance are more active and just the volume of the food they eat allows them to get more nutrients." The heavier girls remained caught in the beauty trap.

A California teenager describes her typical eating pattern. Although she's far from obese, she says that "I struggle daily to control my compulsive eating habits and experience guilt and shame when I fail. I skip breakfast every morning and rarely pack lunches for school. Unfortunately, I usually break down by four o'clock and eat all the junk food I can find. So not only don't I lose weight, but I also tend not to get the nutrition I need. I've tried all the fad diets from Scarsdale to Cambridge along with most of my friends—losing up to five pounds at a time and gaining up to ten back."[12]

Why is losing five or ten pounds important enough to this teenager and her friends that they subject their bodies to such a destructive diet routine? She explains, "Many teenagers [*sic*] feel that they're supposed to look like Brooke Shields or Christie Brinkley; and when they fail to do so, they think that this is some kind of personal flaw or failing." That failure has repercussions elsewhere in their lives. This girl describes often feeling "cheated by life" and a sense of "utter helplessness."

Thirty-year-old Meredith remembers feeling much the same way when she was a teenager. Her obsession with weight became so severe that she ultimately developed life-threatening anorexia nervosa, the self-starvation disease that contributed to the death of singer Karen Carpenter. In recent years, cases of anorexia have been increasing to what some doctors describe as "epidemic proportions." Preston Zucker, M.D., associate clinical professor of pediatrics at Montefiore Hospital and Medical Center, of the Albert Einstein College of Medicine, says that anorexia nervosa may now affect more than 3 percent of our female college population.[13] In addition, Dr. Zucker warns, anorexia has "a 10 to 15 percent mortality rate."

Often we can learn a great deal about our own behavior by examining more extreme forms of it in others. With weight and body image, learning more about anorexia nervosa and bulimia can help us understand our own motivations to control our figures, even though we may never suffer from these disorders ourselves.

Meredith became anorexic during her college years, and she very nearly joined the 10 percent who die as a result of this bizarre mental illness.

As a teenager, Meredith had always been chubby, which caused her a great deal of pain. By the time she was seventeen and had left home for college, "I was about fifteen pounds overweight." That's not a lot, but taken together with her height—Meredith is five feet eight inches—she *felt* huge. "When I was in school, I would hear guys talking about some girl, saying that she had a gorgeous body. The girl was probably five feet one inch and a hundred pounds." The fact that petite girls were popular was certainly not lost on Meredith. "I saw the [more popular] girl as smaller than me, and the only way I could become smaller was to lose weight."

Until she reached college, Meredith had dieted off and on, like most teenage girls, but had never become thin enough to suit herself. "I always felt fat and ugly and left out of things." College was her first experience with living away from home, and she felt under a great deal of pressure to get good grades, make new friends, become a new person. She became ill with what she thought was the flu. "I had it for two weeks and couldn't shake it off. Suddenly I became paralyzed from the waist down and no one could figure out why. I was taken to the hospital."

In the hospital, whether because she was scared half to death by the mysterious paralysis or for some other reason, Meredith simply stopped eating. When she regained the use of her legs and was released from the hospital, she says, "I'd lost weight and, when I looked in the mirror, I liked what I saw." All her life, she'd felt different from other girls, lonely, and "I saw my being alone as a direct result of the way I looked. I didn't realize then that I was shy and introverted and quiet and that *that* was the real reason I was left out."

Meredith treated her weight loss as an omen. If she could just lose enough weight, she was certain that she could be as popular as she'd always hoped. Home from the hospital, she continued to diet. "At first, even my doctor said that it would be good for me, that I should lose weight. But it got out of control. Now, suddenly, the weight was dropping off me—all I had to do was not eat anything. I drank water and black coffee and diet soda with not one calorie."

When she returned to her parents' home, Meredith's new diet habits "instantly became a power struggle with my mother. She would beg me to eat and I would refuse." Meredith had always felt that she couldn't measure up to her mother. "She is always very exact and immaculate and well groomed. She's very poised. She's never been fat. My father used to say to me, 'I wish you would lose weight and look as nice as your mother.' He didn't say that to be malicious, but I took it hard. So now I saw myself as thinner than my mother and it became a big game."

Meredith began to use all of the manipulative methods of the anorexic to get rid of her food. "I would give it to the dog when no one was looking, I would put it down the garbage disposal when I was alone and claim I'd eaten it." For the next seven months, her weight dropped dangerously, until statuesque Meredith weighed only eighty pounds.

Because her weight loss began in 1970, before anorexia became publicized, Meredith's doctors were confused about her illness. Although anorexia nervosa had been described as an eating disorder in medical literature a full hundred years earlier, it was only toward the end of the 1970s that it became widely known.

Meredith's experience is not uncommon among anorexics. They tend to be perfectionists who feel they are under a great deal of pressure from their controlling families. Often they engage in power struggles, particularly with their equally perfectionist mothers. Since they cannot win except by losing—both literally and figuratively—they feel worse and worse about themselves as the disease progresses.

Self-loathing is a common underlying emotion felt by virtually all anorexics. Dr. Raymond E. Vath, a Seattle expert in treating victims of the disease, says, "Because perfection cannot be obtained, feelings of inadequacy and unworthiness lead to an extremely poor self-image."[14] In addition, anorexics often are not happy about being female. They develop a sense of pervasive depression "in which life becomes meaningless, hopeless, overwhelming. It is my opinion that the anorexia is a result of the depression and can be best perceived as a slow form of suicide, much as in alcoholism."

This self-destructive disease starts largely because these women feel that they must be thin (their definition of beauty) in order to be worthwhile. Unless they can look "perfect," they literally don't want to live. Dr. Steven Levenkron, clinical consultant for the Center for the Study of Anorexia Nervosa in New York City and author of *Treating and Overcoming Anorexia Nervosa,* says that the disease "has to be seen as a 'stylistic' breakdown resulting from cultural pressure, since it amounts to a pathological exaggeration of society's message to women. . . . A generation of young girls and women has been indoctrinated by the thin ethic. One has only to review magazine fashion advertisements and television commercials over the past fifteen years to observe the relentless slimming of the models. Epidemiological studies will surely show a parallel between this development and the disorder of emaciation."[15]

In the throes of the disease, anorexics become very manipulative. The disorder becomes, in time, one of their ways of getting attention from their families. Leslie Gershman, who once dropped to seventy pounds during a long battle with anorexia, admits, "You get people wrapped around your little finger. Any time I wanted my father to visit me in the hospital, I knew he'd be there in a second."[16]

Singer Pat Boone's daughter, Cherry Boone O'Neill, says that her siege of anorexia nervosa constituted "four years of constant conflict with my parents over food and weight. Did I eat too little? Had I eaten too much? Did I keep it all down? Had I thrown it up? Had I gained any weight? Did I weigh enough? Did I exercise too much? Had I exercised at all? Was I being honest or was I telling lies?"[17]

O'Neill's adolescent struggles with her weight first began to get out of hand when, as an eighth grader, she stole her mother's diet pills and came close to becoming addicted to them before her thievery was discovered. When she could no longer obtain pills, five-feet-seven-inch Cherry gained weight. By the time she'd reached 140 pounds, she says that her "hatred of fat had escalated into a stark fury and this furious hatred of my fat translated into a furious hatred of myself. That very moment I made a commitment that I was going to shed those ugly pounds regardless of the cost." She soon developed anorexic behavior and her weight dropped to eighty-eight pounds.

Like many anorexics, Cherry Boone O'Neill also had bouts of bulimia—gorging herself with food and then purging either by forcing herself to vomit or by taking large amounts of laxatives and diuretics. Meredith did that, too.

When she had reached eighty pounds, Meredith began eating a little and, she says, "I gained ten pounds in one day. That's known as re-eating edema and it's really water weight. I was terrified to eat when the weight went back on that fast. But then I discovered something else I could do so that I could eat and not gain weight. I bought a package of laxatives in the drugstore and I spent the next twelve years alternating not eating with eating and then purging myself."

Like all anorexics, Meredith has a distorted body image. Even when her weight was at its lowest, she saw a fat person in her mirror.

When she was twenty-one, Meredith got married. "My self image at that time was negative to self-destructive. I got married based on the premise that my husband was the first person who had ever loved me, besides my parents and my sister. I thought that I was stupid and lazy because I was fat and that I was lucky to get anyone to marry me."

The marriage was rocky from the start. "My husband used psychological tactics to control me." Many of his ploys took advantage of her distorted sense of physical appearance. "He would tell me that I was gorgeous, that I had a beautiful body, but then he would compare me unfavorably with somebody else. When I'm thin, I am very thin on top—I have a flat chest. He would tell me that I had no boobs, no sex appeal. My answer to all this was to get thinner. I felt that all my problems would be solved if I could just become beautiful enough and that translated into *thin* enough."

About the time of her wedding, Meredith's laxative purges were no longer working and she once again began gaining weight. Then she found a doctor who would prescribe diuretics to help her drop her water weight gain. "I began abusing them. I took them for six months after I was married and then the worst thing happened. I discovered that I was pregnant and had been for four months."

Like many eating disorder victims, Meredith's menstrual

periods were erratic. When a woman's percentage of body fat is too low, the body rebels and stops its normal functions. Thus, the absence of her periods was not an unusual event for Meredith. That she might be pregnant had not occurred to her.

"I spent the next five months in hell. I was terribly afraid and guilty over what kind of baby might come out of me. I immediately started to eat three healthy meals a day because I was so scared of what I might have done to my baby. When I delivered him, I had no painkilling drugs of any kind—I wasn't going to risk anything else that might harm him. And as far as we can tell, my son has no health problems at all."

It wasn't until her son was nearly eight years old, however, that Meredith had the courage to tell his pediatrician about the diuretics she'd taken early in her pregnancy. "I can't be sure that some health problem that could have been caused by what I was doing won't show up later in his life, so I think the information should be in his medical file."

Meredith's scare didn't change her eating pattern permanently, however. After the baby was born, she went back to her old habits, periods of starvation followed by binging and purging. Her weight would balloon overnight, then drop drastically. Her life resumed its downward spiral. Her marriage broke up, she tried therapy unsuccessfully, and finally, after twelve years of abusing food and her body, she was hospitalized.

When she left the hospital, Meredith finally realized that she needed help, that she had to get over this obsession with food and her weight, if not for her sake, then for her son. She went into therapy and made a concerted effort to get well. She has now managed to control her disease for more than a year. Her weight is higher than she would like it to be: "I weigh 160 now and I feel like I weigh 300." Still, her health is improving and she is determined not to risk ruining it again.

Although a smart woman, Meredith had never appreciated her intelligence. To her, a desirable woman was not brainy but beautiful. These days, however, her goal relies on intelligence rather than on looks. She is completing her doctorate in psychology and intends to become a counselor for other anorexics and bulimics. Her personal ordeal will allow her to give other victims a special kind of understanding and help that she thinks someone who "hasn't been there" cannot provide.

Eating disorders such as anorexia nervosa and bulimia are, of course, the extreme. But many of us can identify with these feelings. Anita B. Siegman, Ph.D., a Los Angeles psychologist specializing in eating disorders, says that "whenever I give a talk to professionals about eating disorders, I will be approached by *all* the female psychologists—this is not an exaggeration. They'll say, 'I'm not anorexic,' or 'I'm not bulimic, but I get crazy like that. If I pig out on Easter Sunday, I feel terrible on Monday,' or 'I feel like I don't want to go out on a date on Saturday if my clothes don't fit right.' So then we begin to talk about how we may be dealing with extremes as therapists, but we have to look at the societal issues and see how they affect us."

A high percentage of victims of these diseases, Dr. Siegman points out, "are women who are somehow overreacting to society's notions of beauty and femininity."

Joel Yaeger, M.D., associate professor of psychiatry and director of the Eating Disorders Clinic at the UCLA Neuropsychiatric Institute, puts the urge to be thin into perspective: "Every society has a way of torturing its women, whether by binding their feet or sticking them into whalebone corsets that are too tight. What contemporary American culture has come up with are tubular designer jeans."[18]

The teenage years are the most common time for anorexia and bulimia to begin, although children as young as eight and women well into middle age also become victims. In a UCLA study of eight hundred bulimics, the average woman said that her eating problems began in her teens as a result of a preoccupation with dieting.[19] Generally by the age of sixteen or seventeen, these women had begun vomiting to rid themselves of food.

Most bulimics, according to Dr. Siegman, who runs several therapy groups for bulimics including one for University of Southern California students, are young women who are very concerned both about physical appearance and about what others think of them. They also tend to throw themselves wholeheartedly into any project they undertake. Such young women may be slightly overweight when they are suddenly struck with the notion that they must reduce. "They go about dieting the same way they go about getting straight A's or being elected to an office in school—with a vengeance. So they end up losing weight very quickly. But, what happens when you lose weight quickly is, first, your metabolic rate slows down and, second, you're going to put [the weight] back on the minute you start eating normally."

While her weight is down, however, the teenager probably receives many compliments on her appearance. "If people are telling you how wonderful you look, it's so seductive that you are willing to pay any price, even at the cost of your health, even at the cost of the whole life-style you've worked so hard to build up." For these young women, what people think of them is what really matters in life. Dr. Siegman says, "I think for all women, no matter how healthy they are, that's [sometimes] the bottom line. I feel that way from time to time, that what really matters is not how I really am but how the world sees me. If you are vulnerable, if you are innocent, if you are inexperienced in life, it's easy to get caught up in that."

According to most experts, both anorexia nervosa and bulimia are increasing rapidly in our slenderness-obsessed society. There are probably more bulimics than anorexics; but because bulimia is a less visible disease (most of its victims are of normal weight), there are no official estimates of the number of women affected. However, within six weeks after he was quoted in a women's magazine article about the eating disorder, Dr. Yaeger received sixteen hundred letters from women who claimed they were bulimic. A program about bulimia broadcast on British television brought ten thousand letters from people seeking help.[20]

A study of more than twelve hundred Chicago high school girls done by Michael Reese Medical Center found, using very conservative criteria, that at least 5 to 8 percent were bulimic. Similar results have been obtained by researchers at the University of Minnesota.[21]

Eating disorders seem to be affecting younger and younger girls. Dr. Fima Lifshitz of North Shore University Hospital in Manhasset, New York, reports that what he calls the "Fear of Obesity Syndrome" is now being documented in prepubescent youngsters.[22] The eating disorder, which possibly is linked to anorexia nervosa, stunts the children's growth and delays puberty. "The children don't eat enough because they fear they will get fat," Dr. Lifshitz says. "And then they hurt themselves . . . they could stunt their growth permanently. They're casualties of this whole slim-and-trim, stay-fit philosophy."

The incidence of eating disorders seems to run higher in certain segments of our population, particularly where physical appearance is of exaggerated importance. Katherine A. Halmi, M.D., a psychiatrist at Cornell University Medical Center in White Plains, New York, found that a full 19 percent of the women at a college concentrating on the performing arts were bulimic.[23]

Suzanne Gordon, author of *Off Balance: The Real World of Ballet,* says that "15 percent of all female dancers and dance students . . . are true anorexics and nearly 50 percent display types of anorexic behavior (crazy diets, sheer starvation, laxative abuse, binge eating and vomiting after eating)."[24] Gordon blames the late George Balanchine for "streamlining the dancer as well as the dance," although she points out that he could not have done so in a society that did not revere unnatural slenderness in females. She describes Balanchine's ideal ballerina: "Breastless, hipless, fast and flexible, the model American ballerina is likely to stand 5-foot-7 and weigh ninety-five pounds."

Eating disorders like anorexia nervosa and bulimia illustrate the extremes to which some women take their obsession with the perfect figure. Both can be health- or life-threatening. Bulimia victims commonly suffer from deterioration of their tooth enamel, sore throats, inflammation of the esophagus, swollen glands, liver damage, nutrition deficiencies, gastric disturbances, and rectal bleeding. In very severe cases, they may suffer rupture of the stomach and disruption of the body's electrolyte and fluid balances, which can cause an irregular heartbeat.

The victim of anorexia also risks rupturing her stomach or esophagus, as well as severe dehydration, gastritis, ulcers, bowel disorders, hypoglycemia, kidney damage, chronic sinusitis, endocrine problems, and abnormal metabolism. In extreme cases, anorexics also suffer severe electrolyte imbalances that might lead to neuromuscular problems, including muscle spasms, cardiac arrest, and death. The late Karen Carpenter, who died of heart failure after a twelve-year battle with anorexia nervosa, was such a case.

There are a variety of analyses of why the current ideal for women is so thin. Kim Chernin, author of *The Obsession: Reflections on the Tyranny of Slenderness,* says that the vogue of thinness reflects men's fear of women's power.[25] When women are clearly subordinate to men, men can delight in womanly figures. But, in times when women are asserting themselves in the male world, "the culture calls for fashions that reflect a distinct male fear of a mature woman's power." A woman's full breasts and natural curves, which "remind men of a time when they depended upon a woman for their very survival," are particularly threatening to men when that woman enjoys economic and political power in addition to traditional "feminine," or motherly, power. Thus, if a woman is powerful, she'd better be thin if she wants to diminish the threat she poses to the men around her.

Chernin also suspects that women, in trying to look more like men (as the female figure becomes thinner, natural curves almost disappear), may be symbolically asking for "the social rights, such as autonomy, that are traditionally reserved for men—much as George Sand wore male attire in order to move freely in masculine society."

Anthropologist Margaret Mackenzie implies that our ambitions of slenderness may reflect new attitudes toward success. "Upwardly mobile women in this era are competing with men, yet most of them are still conditioned to thinking of success personally and professionally in terms of sex and beauty, which are equated with thinness."

There is also the possibility that history is repeating itself. We now have more personal power than ever before, which has triggered a simplification and reduction in the fullness of our clothing. Perhaps we've gone as far as we can in making our clothing scanty and now are trying to take this size reduction one step further by shrinking our bodies. In attempting to become so much thinner than normal, I wonder if we may be compensating for the power—the space—that we've acquired over recent years by taking up less physical space.

We women are often ambivalent about power. We desire power, but we also think that having it makes us "unfeminine." So, if we can concentrate on fulfilling our definition of "superfeminine" (whatever it may be) at the same time we are acquiring power and independence, we are able to feel better about ourselves.

For instance, I remember that in the early seventies I was the only wife and mother in my neighborhood employed outside the home. I wanted my job, my own money, my independence very much. At the same time, I felt rather guilty that I was not conforming to the value system I'd been taught from babyhood. I felt vaguely unfeminine. So I compensated for my "sin" of independence by taking on traditionally feminine tasks with a vengeance. I became the only wife in my neighborhood who drove to the country on autumn weekends, brought home bushels of apples, and canned her own applesauce. I sewed clothes for my son, my husband, and myself. I kept the cookie jar full of homemade cookies. I prided myself on never serving my family mere hamburgers for dinner. *My* meals were far more elaborate. I outhousewifed the housewives. It took me years of constant exhaustion to realize that all that frenetic effort was unnecessary.

My way of being superfeminine in those days did not revolve around my *looks,* but it certainly could have. The principle is the same. Today, the issue of housework is less essential to our feminine self-image. What's left of traditional "femininity" is beauty. If feminine beauty today equals thinness, perhaps at least a part of our fixation on fat reflects our remaining ambivalence over our changing roles.

By spending so much time and effort on our diets, on our exercise programs, on what we believe to be the most easily controlled aspect of physical beauty, we may well be trying to reassure ourselves that we're still women after all. Yet, we're making it harder to escape from the beauty trap.

We also must realize that few of us ever truly achieve our weight and figure goals, at least not for long. It is far easier to make and can thirty quarts of applesauce over a weekend than it is to achieve and maintain the perfect body—particularly when the ideal figure is unnaturally slender.

So, most of us, because we set up unachievable goals for ourselves, end up failing, and thus doing additional damage to our already-battered self-esteem.

We do have certain payoffs, however, in being obsessed

with body weight. For instance, by being compulsive about fat and dieting, we are in tune with much of our society. The fat fixation carries chic social respectability these days. A popular topic of conversation in any women's group is weight loss and figure control, to the point where, as one woman said, she's embarrassed to admit to friends that she's *not* on a diet.

Unfortunately, many of us have inflated expectations about what a perfect figure will do for us. We may believe that as soon as we find the right diet and the right motivation, all the problems in our lives magically will be solved. If we only looked "right," we tell ourselves, we'd be popular, sexy, successful, rich, whatever we lack in our lives. Believing this myth allows us to concentrate all our efforts on one goal—losing weight. Our figure becomes the target for all our worries, disappointments, ambitions. Unfortunately, having a gorgeous body simply won't solve all our problems. (In fact, because having a lovely figure increases the chance of being treated as a sex object, a great body may simply create a new and different kind of problem.) Dr. Siegman often faces the results of these shattered expectations among her bulimic clients. "A large segment of the women who come to me for therapy decided to do so when they reached their ideal weight and were still miserable." Their dreams did not automatically come true when the scale dropped to that magic number.

Being obsessed with our bodies also allows us to postpone various goals, sometimes indefinitely. Most of us have told ourselves many times, "As soon as I lose ten pounds, I'll . . ." Just what we will do when we've lost that ten pounds (or twenty or fifty) might be look for a better job, take a trip, go back to school, find a husband, have a baby, virtually anything that takes some effort. We are able to postpone that resolution, *to avoid taking either action or risks,* as long as we fail to lose weight. Our weight and diet become a wonderful excuse for our passivity.

Of course, if we spend an inordinate amount of time failing to achieve a perfect, fat-free body, we can feel quite sorry for ourselves. Self-pity seems to be seductive to many weight-obsessed people, even though it's generally very unattractive to those around them. Sometimes, by demonstrating enough self-pity, we even cajole others into feeling sorry for us. We attract attention, even if it's completely negative attention.

If we really intend to live happy, profitable lives, however, we have to stop using the fat fixation as an excuse for not doing so. The fact is, we are not fettered nearly so much by our extra pounds as we are by our beauty trap minds.

10

THE BEAUTY SCULPTORS

In 1972, actress-singer-dancer Ann-Margret's career began to take a sharp turn for the better.[1] Her beauty had always gained her attention, but with her recent Academy Award nomination for her role in *Carnal Knowledge,* she was finally beginning to be appreciated as a serious actress as well. Her successful Nevada nightclub act was drawing larger crowds at every show. Ann-Margret's professional life was brimming with promise.

She was preparing for her nightclub act on a fateful September day, rehearsing on a twenty-two-foot-high platform above the stage at Lake Tahoe's Sahara Hotel. Suddenly the scaffolding collapsed and Ann-Margret was hurled to the ground, landing with an impact that crushed the left side of her beautiful face and fractured both her jaw and her left arm. In one horrible moment, her promising career, and possibly her life, were seriously jeopardized.

She was unconscious for four days. "When I opened my eyes in that hospital room and nobody would give me a mirror, I knew how awful I looked," Ann-Margret says. It didn't take her long to put her disfigurement into perspective, however. "It didn't matter. Nothing mattered except that I was alive. I was ugly, I hurt all over, but I was ecstatic."

The accident occurred at a particularly turbulent time in her life. Ann-Margret's father had been hospitalized with cancer and part of her concern over her own condition was that it would upset him. She felt that she should set an example for her father, that she could raise his spirits by proving she would recover and resume her career. So, while Ann-Margret was grateful simply for living through the freak accident, she was also thankful that plastic surgeons were able to repair her face. Without their help, she might never have appeared on a stage or in a film again.

Ann-Margret's painful reconstructive surgery took weeks, during which her father's condition worsened. She was determined to keep up his morale, however, so "as each of my bandages was removed, I'd go hobbling into his hospital room. My jaw was still wired and I could hardly talk—God, it was frustrating—but I'd stand there and say, 'Daddy, you watch! I'll be back on that stage in November, you hear? You just watch!' "

Thanks both to her own courage and determination, and to her surgeons' skill, Ann-Margret kept her promise. Two thousand people cheered her as she sang her father's favorite song, "When You're Smiling," at her Las Vegas Hilton comeback. Terminally ill, Ann-Margret's father watched his daughter's performance over closed-circuit television in his hospital room.

Today, Ann-Margret suffers an occasional click when she closes her jaw, and she's still aware of the accident's physical and emotional effects. But no one else can see them when they watch her perform. Without the skill of reconstructive surgery, her comeback might have been impossible.

Like Ann-Margret, many women have had occasion to feel grateful for the reconstructive expertise of modern medicine. We may be able to diet off pounds, to make up our faces, to dress attractively, but there are some changes we can't make by ourselves. We can't rebuild a face crushed in an accident, replace a breast lost to cancer, repair an acne-scarred complexion, remove wrinkles and sags from an aging face, or pare down a bump on a nose. For these improvements, some of us are willing to explore and submit to a variety of medical techniques, including surgery. We consider the inherent risks less important than the potential gains.

For Ann-Margret, whose career depends in part upon her physical beauty, it's easy to understand that the plastic surgeon's techniques are vital. Indeed, for any woman disfigured either by a congenital defect or by accident, plastic surgery can perform miracles. With the help of modern medicine, she can hope to lead a normal life.

Luckily, these techniques are continually improving. Half a century ago, a woman who had suffered a fall like Ann-Margret's literally would have been changed overnight from an envied beauty into an object of pity. Medical science would not have been able to help.

Former French test pilot Jacqueline Auriol, who is now on the board of directors of Avon-France, was one of the first to benefit from reconstructive surgery techniques.[2] In July of 1949, Auriol was piloting a test plane over the Seine River. "I had the impression that the plane was much too low and then, suddenly, saw nothing more, felt nothing more," she says. The plane crashed and Jacqueline Auriol was slammed, face first, into the instrument panel. "I had no face anymore and I didn't even know it," she wrote later of the crash. Her cheekbones and jawbones were crushed, her nose was gone, her eye sockets were fractured—her entire face was flattened.

At the time of the crash, Auriol, whose father-in-law, Victor Auriol, was the president of France, was on a round of official engagements. Her position in French society was highly visible and a newspaper recently had termed her "the prettiest woman in Paris." Suddenly, she looked like a freak.

"When you live in a world where everyone's eyes are

evenly placed on both sides of a nose, you know you are different when you have no nose and your eyeballs roll down your cheeks," she says. Her other injuries, broken ribs and a fractured collarbone, healed, but her face required a miracle.

It took years, but Jacqueline Auriol finally found her miracle. At first her quest was simply to find a way to look human. In 1949, regaining her beauty seemed beyond hope. Auriol became a beautiful woman again, but the face she acquired was not the one she had had before her accident. When she peered into the mirror after her series of reconstructive surgeries, she confronted an unfamiliar face. She would wear this "manmade face" for the rest of her life.

The man who gave Jacqueline Auriol her new face was the pioneering American plastic surgeon John Marquis Converse of New York University Medical Center. In 1982, Auriol returned to New York City to help honor the memory of the late Dr. Converse, who "played such an important part in my life." She delivered a corporate donation to help fund the $1 million John Marquis Converse Chair of Plastic Surgery Research at New York University Medical Center.

A woman equally as courageous as Ann-Margret, Jacqueline Auriol says that she's never been bitter about her accident. In fact, "I was lucky to have that crash." It changed her life. With her face destroyed, she no longer appeared at official functions for her father-in-law. As a result, she had time to reflect upon her life. She decided that she was going to "get even" with flying. "In the hospital, I determined that it was necessary for me to begin a new life in aviation."

After her recuperation from her many operations, Auriol pursued her dream, becoming a full-fledged test pilot and later the first woman to crack the sound barrier in a plane in level flight. (The late American pilot Jacqueline Cochran is credited as the first woman to fly faster than the speed of sound. However, Auriol notes that the Cochran plane was in a dive when it broke the sound barrier, thus its speed was increased by gravity.)

Now in her mid-sixties, Auriol flew until she was fifty-four. She has also worked as an interior decorator for an airline and a hotel chain, in addition to her board position for Avon. Without her new face, few of her accomplishments since 1949 would have been possible.

Fortunately, of course, most of us will never have to have a new face constructed by the surgeon's scalpel. What's more likely is that we will someday consider having a new breast constructed to replace one lost to cancer. Statistics show that one American woman in every nine will contract breast cancer during her lifetime. Most of these women will undergo a mastectomy as a result, causing both physical and psychological mutilation. Losing a breast, for many women, means losing an essential part of their femininity and beauty.

One mastectomy patient said, "Once an uninhibited person, I was afraid. I kept thinking, 'What if men who admired my body from afar found out that I was a fraud? Would others laugh and joke if they saw my lopsided body?' "

Betty Rollin, author of *First You Cry,* a book about her emotional reaction to her own mastectomy, wrote of planning a quick trip to her corner market, something that required her to conceal the flat side of her chest because she "couldn't face the possibility of shocking and repulsing my fellow shoppers. In America, bodies are whole, teeth are straight, and the sight of a deformed person—that's you kid—is a turnoff. It's unpatriotic to be a freak."[3]

Dr. Brenda Solomon of the Chicago Institute for Psychoanalysis says that "it's very difficult to undergo surgery that mutilates any part of the body—particularly a sexual part of the body."[4]

When Californian Norma Hertzog had her mastectomy in 1981, she had already determined that she would undergo breast reconstruction several months later. Although that knowledge helped her face the original surgery, the six months between the mastectomy and the reconstruction were difficult.

An energetic woman in her early fifties, Hertzog is a member of the Costa Mesa City Council and owns and manages two developmental preschools as well. She has never been the type to let illness interrupt her hectic schedule. Even after her cancer surgery, she was back on her feet and working within two weeks.

One of her first appointments after the surgery was to give a speech. "I thought, 'I'll just go to a store and buy a falsie.' " She remembered that when she was younger (and when larger breasts were more fashionable) "falsies" were readily available in lingerie departments. But times had changed. "I went everywhere and I guess they just don't make falsies anymore." All she could find was a $160 prosthesis and that was the wrong size. Her speaking engagement was less than two days away and her clothes hung oddly on her right side.

"I just couldn't go like *that.*" Almost in tears, she called a friend who works with a breast center. Luckily, a woman who had undergone reconstruction had just turned in two 34B breast forms—Hertzog's size. She borrowed them and "as soon as I had my own reconstruction, I brought them back so somebody else could use them."

Because Norma Hertzog knew that it was only a matter of a few months before her new breast would be created surgically, she was reluctant to spend a large amount of money to be fitted with her own prosthesis, which is held securely in a pocket inside a special bra. Her frugality soon led to an amusing if embarrassing situation. Hertzog was working in one of her preschools, energetically scrubbing a tabletop, when her borrowed prosthesis suddenly popped out of her bra, slid down her right arm, and dropped onto the floor. Alone in the room, she made a dive for the breast form and was frantically trying to stuff it back up her sleeve and into her bra when one of the teachers entered the room. "She stared at me and asked, 'What are you doing?' " Hertzog recalls with a hearty laugh. "I said, 'What does it look like I'm doing? I'm putting my boob back!' We just stood there and howled."

Hertzog, a tall, attractive blonde with an infectious smile, has a habit of looking for the humor in every situation, no matter how grim. She describes her first thought when, shortly after her mastectomy, she worked up the courage to look at what remained of her chest: "This is the only blank wall I've ever seen that could be improved with graffiti." The idea struck her funny and she laughed until the tears rolled down her face, her typical way of releasing emotional tension.

Yet, as it would be for any woman, Hertzog's surgery was traumatic. She found her body image greatly altered and, as a divorced woman, she was particularly worried about how men would react to her disfigurement. "I think that it really helped to know that that condition was only temporary."

Before she had her reconstruction, she "was just plain uncomfortable. No matter what I put on, there was one decent side and the other side just hung. I would always put on a bra," even when she was just sitting around the house, "because sometimes my kids would have company and I'd have my housecoat on." Like author Betty Rollin, she didn't want to upset anyone by calling attention to her mastectomy.

Her frequent travel to business conferences created another problem. Often Hertzog would have to share a hotel room with another woman and "I really didn't want my roommates to see my scars." She felt that her body would frighten or repulse them.

After waiting to heal completely from the mastectomy and to make sure that no new cancer cells were discovered, Norma Hertzog tried a new kind of breast reconstruction surgery. Her procedure combined a "tummy tuck" operation with the creation of her new breast. The operation involved taking skin and muscle from her abdominal area, then building a tunnel to the chest and drawing abdominal tissue through it to form her new breast. The result was a new breast constructed entirely of material from Hertzog's own body. Unlike other reconstruction techniques, Hertzog's required no silicone implant to form the breast shape.

Before her reconstructive surgery, Hertzog preferred to hide her body, but after the operation, she says, she "wanted everyone to see because I felt whole again." She has told her story in speeches, in print, and on television in hopes of helping other women realize that life does go on following a cancer diagnosis.

A woman's sense of her physical appearance, she believes, is a critical factor in the treatment of breast cancer. Many women believe that if they have a mastectomy, they will lose their feminine beauty and become repulsive to others. So they either don't look for the early signs of breast cancer or they ignore them. As a result, too many die needlessly.

A reconstructed breast, sometimes called a "breast mound," is not identical to an original breast. Hertzog is adamant that breast reconstruction is not cosmetic surgery. "I actually had a woman tell me that my reconstruction was just cosmetic surgery!" she says indignantly. "I thought I would go through the roof. I said, 'The first time you have *your* breast removed, come and tell me that's cosmetic surgery.' I told her, 'If you want to see the scars on my chest, I'll be glad to show them to you.' It's not pleasant and it's *not* cosmetic surgery."

Not all women who undergo mastectomy opt for reconstruction. Much depends upon their body image, age, marital status, and other factors. Some don't feel that undergoing a second major (and expensive) operation is justified. Others simply adjust more quickly to the loss of a breast. In fact, one woman wrote a magazine article about her decision to appear one-breasted—not to wear a prosthesis—after her mastectomy, even while swimming in mixed company.[5] Most women don't possess that self-confidence, however. Reconstruction might help them feel attractive again and accelerate their readjustment to life after surgery.

Most women who choose reconstruction are pleased with having made that choice, according to Shirley Devol-VanLieu, Ph.D., who conducted in-depth interviews with twenty-four such women for her doctoral dissertation in social work at the University of Southern California. Only one woman in her sample (who had encountered serious medical problems with her implant) was so dissatisfied that she would not choose to have breast reconstruction again.

An advantage for women facing this kind of surgery, Dr. Devol-VanLieu believes, would be "talking to other women who've been through it." The term "breast construction" is misleading. "What is constructed is not a breast. Some women said they heard the word 'mound' but still expected 'a real breast.' Almost all of the women who did not feel well informed wanted to see and/or talk to a woman who had completed the procedure." A woman's adjustment to her reconstructed breast is made easier, Dr. Devol-VanLieu learned, if she can actually see and touch one before her own surgery.

Dr. Devol-VanLieu found that mastectomy and reconstruction exerted profound influence on each woman's feelings of attractiveness. The women she questioned "felt attractive before the mastectomy, less so afterwards. Their self-esteem increased after the reconstruction, but not to the former level."

Norma Hertzog agrees. "When you get to be over fifty, as I am, your body is not the same as it was at twenty-five or thirty. But two years ago [before her mastectomy] it was a lot nicer than it is now." Without surgery, however, she might not have lived those two years. With the reconstruction, she no longer is reminded constantly of her battle with cancer.

Losing a breast is only one of many physically disfiguring conditions that can so reduce a woman's quality of life that she actually questions whether or not she wants to continue living. We'd all like to believe that no specific lack of beauty is that important, but to many women, it is.

New Yorker Patty Fischer, who was a victim of severe recalcitrant cystic acne, often felt that way.[6] Her face was a constant mass of pus-filled eruptions. "I looked like a freak," she says. "People on the street made comments. I got to the point where I didn't want to live anymore. The idea of death was always on my mind."

Patty Fischer enjoyed an ideal high school life—plenty of dates, a role in a school play, a place on the cheerleading squad—until she turned sixteen. Then the disease, which is often permanently disfiguring and affects the neck and back as well as the face, struck her. She and her mother began a discouraging round of appointments with dermatologists. For the next seven years, Fischer tried various acne treatments, including drugs, sulfa packs, and painful injections. "I was in pain if someone touched my face or accidently brushed against it," she recalls.

In despair, Fischer was finally accepted into an experimental treatment program at the State University of New York Downstate Medical Center in Brooklyn. She was treated with Accutane, a synthetic derivative of vitamin A, over a five-month period. At the end of that time, she says, "I didn't have one cyst left." Her life once again became worth living.

Accutane treatment can have sometimes severe side effects, including chapped lips, dry skin, muscle cramps, and temporary thinning of the hair. It has caused birth defects in laboratory animals, so it cannot be used by pregnant women. For Patty Fischer, the side effects were a small price to pay to rid herself of her severe acne condition. Following the drug treatment, she continued in the experimental program so that scar tissue left by her acne could be removed. There are a variety of new medical techniques for removing acne scars, such as dermabrasion and collagen injections, but they cannot be used until the disease is arrested.

Although living with an inflamed and scarred face is certainly possible, for Patty Fischer, it wasn't worth the emotional pain. She couldn't abide the curious stares, the feeling that she was repulsive to others, her lack of a love life, or the idea of living this way forever. Fortunately, medical science had developed a technique for restoring her attractive appearance.

Not all women who seek out medical doctors to improve their appearance are correcting birth defects or the results of accidents and illnesses, of course. Much more common is a desire to improve upon something that's far from truly debilitating. They want their noses shortened, their breasts enlarged, their wrinkles removed, their abdomens flattened. More women seek these surgical improvements each year.

Since 1970—ironically, at the height of the Women's Movement—the number of cosmetic surgeries performed each year has more than doubled. This trend has resulted in startling statistics: Some four thousand surgeons, as well as hundreds of doctors not trained in plastic surgery techniques, are now in the medical and surgical beautification business. They earn a total of four billion dollars each year, some doctors as much as a million dollars each. A million and a half Americans (both women and men) annually opt for trying to improve their looks with face-lifts, eyelid tucks, breast augmentations, and similar operations.

One effect of the increased popularity of cosmetic surgery is that people who've had such operations are no longer keeping it a secret. When former first lady Betty Ford had a face-lift in 1978, she announced candidly, "I'm sixty years old and I wanted a nice new face to go with my beautiful new life."[7] Phyllis Diller has admitted having an eye-lift, face-lift, and breast reduction. Cher owns up to having had plastic surgery on her face and breasts.

When "before and after" photographs of Miss America of 1982, Debra Sue Maffett, surfaced in the press, she admitted that she had surgery on her nose prior to winning her title, although she claims the surgery was to correct a "breathing disorder."

In 1983 Carol Burnett spoke openly with several national publications about surgery that improved her profile, adding about four millimeters to her chin and correcting what she calls "the Burnett lower lip." Never one to take herself too seriously, Burnett says that "the greatest thing of all" is her new ability to feel "the rain on my chin for the first time."[8] She also admits that she feels much prettier.

Actress Mariel Hemingway had breast implant surgery before starring as the late actress Dorothy Stratten in *Star 80*.[9] She claims, however, that she would have had the surgery anyway. "I thought about it very carefully before I did it. Nobody in our family has much of a bust. But I decided I didn't want to go through life being looked on as just an athletic tomboy.

"All my life I've felt feminine inside. But growing up in a place like Idaho and not being around feminine women much, I guess I did develop into a tomboy. I liked dressing up, but nobody much did it there, so I just forgot about it. Now, since making this movie, I feel I've become a real woman and I like it."

The great increase in cosmetic surgery testifies to our growing concern over our appearance. (This concern is hardly limited to either women or Americans. A California cosmetic surgeon says that at least half of her patients are men. Even in China, where cosmetic surgery was once banned as bourgeois Western decadence, at least one surgeon is earning a high income performing an average of fifteen "eye jobs" a month, to create more Westernized eyelids for his Asian customers. The surgeon displays a photograph of Sophia Loren in his office.)

Los Angeles cosmetic surgeon E. Michael Molnar says that "competition for the good things in life is getting more severe. People have to put themselves in the best possible position, and physical beauty becomes an extremely important edge."[10]

Yet surgery can do only so much. A smaller nose, fewer wrinkles, a more prominent chin won't change a woman's life. "Don't look for surgery to repair a broken romance, or as a diversion after grief, or to find a new job after being fired," advises Dr. John A. Grossman of General Rose Memorial Hospital in Denver.[11] "Your motivation should be directed toward a particular feature which you don't like and have *not* liked for some time."

Los Angeles psychologist Patricia Keith-Spiegel points out that many women are dissatisfied with the results of cosmetic surgery, not because their physical changes are disappointing, but because the life changes for which they irrationally had hoped are not forthcoming. Before surgery, many women may convince themselves that having a face-lift will gain them a husband or that removal of the "saddlebags" on their hips will result in greater career success. In most cases, finding a husband and succeeding on the job have little or no connection with an aging face or more-than-ample hips. They have more to do with personality, effort, intelligence, self-confidence. So the surgery doesn't—in fact, couldn't possibly—have the desired results. In the end, Dr. Keith-Spiegel says, the major result of some cosmetic surgery may well be depression.

A good plastic surgeon will attempt to determine a patient's motivation for surgery and reject those with unrealistic expectations. Los Angeles cosmetic surgeon Dr. Ronald Strahan says he rejects one patient in twenty for this reason.[12] "I have to determine whether the patient has realistic goals. If the patient is an actor, I have to be sure he understands that just because I remove a bump from his nose that it is no guarantee that parts will come rolling in."

Changing our features might even be guilt-producing. One woman in her late twenties, for example, had always disliked her receding chin and wanted to have it built up surgically. She was afraid to do it while her mother, who had the same kind of chin, was alive, fearing her mother would take it as a symbolic rejection. So the daughter waited until her mother died before scheduling her operation.

In another case, a young wife, who had her nose surgically altered as a teenager, didn't tell her husband about the operation until she was forced to, after their first child was born. The baby had an unusually large nose, and the husband had begun to harbor doubts about whether he was really the child's biological father.

Unlike breast reconstructions, elective surgery for purely cosmetic reasons is often not covered by medical insurance. A simple face-lift, for example, costs from $2,000 to more than $5,000. Removal of pockets of fat from the body can cost $3,000. Reshaping a nose may cost $2,000. The addition of hospital charges can double these costs, and most cosmetic surgeons require cash in advance.

Many of these procedures carry with them the risks and pain inherent in any major surgery, too. For instance, an abdominoplasty, commonly known as a "tummy tuck," is performed under general anesthesia, which occasionally causes heart failure. The operation also sometimes requires blood transfusions. Dr. Robert Spence, assistant professor of plastic surgery at the University of Maryland, warns prospective patients, "It is less painful than internal organ surgery because it does not cut through muscle, but it can take a long time to heal, and you can have a pulling sensation and numbness for months."[13]

Also, in many of the body contouring surgeries, prominent scars result. Surgical thigh reduction, for instance, can leave the patient with legs that are pleasingly shaped but noticeably scarred. "You are trading one significant deformity for another significant deformity," says Dr. Spence.

He adds other dangers of surgical fat removal and body contouring: The repositioned skin, because it is moved far from its source of blood in this type of surgery, might die. The wound could become infected. A patient can hemorrhage. And, bedbound after surgery, she might get thrombophlebitis.

Prospective plastic surgery patients should be aware of the many disfiguring and dangerous problems caused by unskilled surgeons who have infiltrated the practice because of the money to be made. Breast implants have turned rock hard and some have been suspected of causing cancer. Botched nose jobs have cost patients their sense of smell or left them with noses pared to virtual nonexistence. Poor face-lifts have left facial nerves cut, so that one side of the face is asymmetrical and without expression. Many of these procedures have resulted in serious infections and ugly scars. Some patients have died.

Plastic surgery and other medical techniques can perform miracles both physically and psychologically for truly disfigured women. Medicine can provide a new lease on life, restore self-esteem, make us look and feel normal again.

For those of us with less severe beauty problems, competent plastic surgery can be beneficial as well. Having such surgery is certainly nothing to be ashamed of. As Los Angeles psychotherapist Laura Schlessinger, an attractive woman in her thirties, says, "If my face falls three inches (someday), I'll have it hiked up. Why not?"

But skin care expert Irma Shorell, who is the daughter of a plastic surgeon, warns women about being "too greedy."[14] She advises not having a face-lift too early in life. In her late fifties, Shorell says that she's never had plastic surgery: "I'll postpone it until there's nothing else I can do about the sagging and bagging." In contrast, I know several women who had face-lifts while they were still in their thirties and now, in their forties, are facing a decision to have another.

In today's beauty-conscious climate, there's also a very real danger that cosmetic surgery may come to seem almost a *requirement* for women of a certain age. In many circles, it's a fad to have *something* surgically altered. I've noticed several magazine articles recently that purport to give readers a timetable for each of several face-lifts they might expect to have during their lifetimes.

In 1983, one of Los Angeles's largest department store chains held a series of beauty conferences for its customers, featuring seminars on cosmetic surgery. At these seminars, shoppers were invited to "meet the most highly trained plastic and reconstructive surgeons in California" and "enjoy a slide presentation featuring before and after surgery results." Today, plastic surgery is being marketed as casually as a new fall wardrobe.

This kind of pressure to make medical and surgical alterations as a matter of course can have severely detrimental effects on our self-esteem, our physical health, and our financial status.

Clearly, no woman should let herself be coerced into making any change in her appearance, least of all one that requires her to submit to expensive and possibly dangerous elective surgery.

There's nothing wrong with our being satisfied with a less-than-perfect nose, a pear-shaped body, or every one of the wrinkles we "earn" as we grow older. Self-acceptance is a sign of mental health, a sign of proper perspective, a sign of freedom from the beauty trap.

If we can become more self-accepting, more able to get on with the rest of our lives successfully after having protruding ears pinned back or uncomfortably large breasts reduced or any other realistic medical procedure, fine. The main danger we face lies in our expecting that, once the surgeon's scalpel awards us a changed appearance, our newfound beauty will *by itself* enrich our lives.

The main danger lies in our beauty trap thinking.

11

PRETTY AS A PICTURE

One woman might envy Jane Pauley's hair. Another might dream of having a figure like Cheryl Tiegs's, eyes like Elizabeth Taylor's, or a creamy complexion like that of the model on the cover of this month's issue of *Glamour.*

Each of us carries a picture in our heads of the way we'd like to look, if only nature had been kinder or artifice more successful. Chances are that this picture resembles the beautiful women so prevalent in the media—the actresses, television reporters, and models who entertain us, inform us, and try to sell us products.

We would do well to remember that beauty is a commodity and, as such, it's sold to us constantly, both directly and indirectly. The concept we've been taught from infancy, that much of our feminine value is in our beauty, is reinforced for us daily by the communications media. Each time we turn on the television set or open a magazine or glance through a department store catalog or go to a movie, we are confronted with a preponderance of beautiful women. Hardly any of them are overweight, or have pimples, or are obviously older than thirty-five. The gorgeous women the media display—the ones with the perfect noses, the straight teeth, the latest hairdos, and the thin bodies—become the norm against which we all learn to measure ourselves. We don't compare ourselves (comparison somehow always seems to creep into our self-assessments) with the colleague in the next office or the neighbor who lives across the street. We try to measure up to Christie Brinkley or Joan Lunden. Not surprisingly, most of us lose in that kind of contest.

Psychologist Ellen Berscheid says that our increasing concern about beauty may in part be because of "the larger role the media play in our lives. Hollywood has always worshiped beauty, but now television holds before us twenty-four hours a day, every day, an extraordinarily high standard of physical attractiveness—one that may be too high, incidentally, for most people to achieve."[1]

Once we have bought the idea that beautiful is best, we become vulnerable to a more direct sales pitch, the one that exploits our desire to be beautiful (and, by extension, our desire to be happy) and that sells us products and services. They range from products that relate directly to beauty—makeup, foundation garments, diet foods, clothing, hairstyling services, health spa memberships—to virtually any product that we can be seduced into buying because we want to look, and be, like the pretty female who advertises it.

Images represented in the media begin to influence us very early in life. Los Angeles psychologist Michael Doyle notes that young children watch many hours of television each day (often far more than adults do) and "you don't have to watch too much TV to see what's being communicated. . . . The subtleties of the message [include] how women are dressed, and what kinds of women get on TV as opposed to the kinds of men. I think the message is real clear that physical attractiveness is a crucial dimension for women."

According to Dr. Doyle, television commercials, in particular, have a big impact on youngsters. "If you observe a child closely, she will be rather passive during the show and you can see an elevation of her interest during the commercials. They're designed to grab attention—the noise level, the music, the visual imagery rapidly changing."

By the age of fourteen, the average child has viewed 350,000 television commercials. Those commercials, as well as the entertainment programs kids watch, often feature children, and when they're females, they're undoubtedly *pretty* little girls. Occasionally a boy actor can be less than perfect-looking—splashed with freckles, slightly chubby, or missing his front teeth. Yet girls on television or modeling in magazines and catalogs are expected to be attractive.

Talent agent Jeannette Walton, of Hollywood's Wormser, Helfand and Joseph, Inc., says that good looks are vital for the child models and actresses her agency represents. If a department store is putting together a catalog, for instance, "their first requisite in most instances is beauty. They want beautiful, all-American children." Occasionally, stores will include a minority or ethnic child in an ad layout, "but they want beautiful ethnics."

For some ads and commercials, such as those selling cereals, classic beauty becomes less important, she adds. Child models featured in those ads, particularly boys, can be "personality kids. The Norman Rockwell concept is very big."

The children who are represented by an agency like Wormser, Helfand and Joseph are sometimes as young as a few months old and, if their looks fit into the prescribed category and they are well behaved, they can expect to work until they reach their awkward teen-age years. The more successful children, after a hiatus, might return to modeling around age eighteen and continue indefinitely. They learn at an early age that their beauty is a commodity that they can sell to advertisers and that advertisers can sell to consumers.

It's the summer of 1983, and several hundred aspiring models are gathered at the Waldorf-Astoria Hotel in New York City for the International Talent Modeling Schools and

Agencies convention. All shapes and sizes, the young women range in height from perhaps five feet two to five feet eleven and in weight from under 100 to more than 150 pounds.

At this convention, the participants, all modeling school graduates, have an opportunity to be judged by representatives of model agencies from the United States, Europe, and Japan. A lucky few will be signed to contracts. The rest will go home and revise their dreams.

An eighteen-year-old honey blonde from Indianapolis, Indiana, waits in line patiently for a chance to show her pictures to a representative of the Wilhemina Agency, one of New York's largest. Her dream of becoming the next Christie Brinkley or Cheryl Tiegs is dimming as the convention progresses.

Slender and pretty but not classically beautiful, this young woman, at five feet seven, is barely tall enough to be a fashion model. More important than her lack of height is that she just doesn't have this year's "look." Perhaps, she thinks, the problem is her hair. It's curly and bouncy, a bit on the short side as compared with the New York models' tresses. She decides that it's "too Indianapolis," so she's going to have it restyled.

Yesterday, she tells me, disappointment clouding her features, she interviewed with another model agency's representative. "The lady took one look at my photos and said, 'You're a commercial model, not a high fashion model.' I want to be a high fashion model. I want to do runway work. *I want it so bad.*" She has had a little runway experience back in Indiana, "but Indianapolis is nothing like *this.*"

She's hardly alone in desiring this particular career. She's surrounded by young women from towns all over the country, pretty females wearing their best dresses, their hair carefully curled, their makeup expertly applied. Only a handful are stunningly beautiful, but they all share the dream of model stardom. They've all spent their time and money attending modeling schools. Possibly *one* of them will make it to the top echelons of modeling, if she's very lucky.

In this business, agents claim that they can tell instantly whether or not a model has "it," that special but indefinable quality that ensures that a model is successful. Weight can be gained or lost, hairdos can be changed, makeup can be applied, but none of these characteristics will give a girl "it" if she hasn't had it from birth. Yet hope springs eternal. As the young woman from Indianapolis moves ahead in the line, a tall redhead with heavy thighs scurries down the hotel corridor, excitedly calling to a friend, "They asked me to come back in a bathing suit!"

John Casablancas, founder and president of Elite Model Management, one of the three largest model agencies in the world, says that his agency interviews about sixty thousand aspiring models each year. From that number, perhaps five hundred or six hundred are signed to contracts and, a year later, only a third of them are still modeling. It's a very tough business to crack and an even tougher one in which to become successful.

The head of Los Angeles's largest fashion model agency, Nina Blanchard, says that statistically, it's easier to be elected to the United States Congress than to become a top high fashion model. "I get 400 phone calls a day and 5,000 pieces of mail each week. From these I might find one picture that I consider right for my agency. Many of the kids don't even fit the most basic physical requirements."[2]

Those requirements are quite specific. John Casablancas says that an American model must be at least five feet seven inches tall but not more than six feet. The Paris model must be taller, five feet eight or five feet nine inches, but in Japan a Caucasian model who's only five feet six inches could do well. Since the camera adds pounds, models must be thin, yet not appear skinny. And they must keep their weight down. A few extra pounds or sleepless nights, and their "look" fades.

This comparative handful of elite women who work as models becomes the norm for all of us. Too often, we feel negative about ourselves because we can't manage to be physical clones of these young women, whose beauty fits an extremely narrow definition and who are willing to work constantly to maintain it.

The models who make it, of course, appear to have everything that women are taught to want: beauty, glamour, money, fame. Superstar model Christie Brinkley, for example, earns roughly $350,000 a year posing for Cover Girl cosmetics and doing other product endorsements.[3] With the addition of her exercise book, numerous other modeling assignments, a film role, and royalties from her posters, she's become virtually an industry unto herself.

A career like Brinkley's is precisely what all those young women from Indianapolis or Little Rock or Bozeman or Miami visualize. Because they yearn to be star models, they are frequently victimized, particularly when they leave home to follow their dreams to New York or Los Angeles or Paris. Nina Blanchard meets them frequently. "These street kids blow into Hollywood and have no idea that this town is just full of scams. If someone says to a fifteen-year-old, 'Hey, stick with me, I can make you a star,' the kid is going to believe them precisely because they want it so badly. I'll tell you, sometimes I feel so frustrated with them that I just want to grab them and shake some sense into them."

Some of the hopefuls return home filled with disillusionment. The less fortunate end up in prostitution.

The handful who manage to begin a modeling career discover that the actual work is at variance with their fantasy. It's hardly all glamour, even for the supermodels. They live under constant pressure and difficult conditions. Because of magazine publishers' lead times, for instance, they're likely to find themselves modeling bathing suits in forty-degree weather or fur coats in a heat wave. They may travel all night for an early morning photography session. Yet models are expected to look as though they're always completely fresh and rested. Their careers are short-lived. Successful fashion models last ten years at best. During that time, if they're smart, they're planning financially for an early retirement.

Fewer than twelve hundred women are represented by New York's modeling agencies and they earn an average of $30 thousand a year.[4] Only about twenty-five earn the $300 thousand or more that's often touted in the press.

John Casablancas (whose agency has offices in New York, Chicago, Los Angeles, Dallas, London, Paris, Tokyo, Munich, and Hamburg) says that getting started in modeling, even for a woman who has the right look, is very difficult. "There are some models who make five hundred a month. I know some kids who've made nothing for three, four months, not one booking. It takes a lot of guts at the beginning. You have to be very tough."

New models spend months on "go-sees," which is the industry's term for auditions. They work for minimum hourly rates at first as they build their books of photographs. They meet constant rejection. When she's rejected time after time because she doesn't *look* right, it can be very difficult for a young woman to maintain her self-confidence. Because they tend to be young, without much experience in life, many of them can't take the pressure.

Linda Bean told a *Boston Globe* reporter about her trying year as a Paris model.[5] Bean met other young women like herself crossing the Atlantic to enter this highly competitive world. Many of them quickly discovered French cooking, Bean said, and gained ten or fifteen pounds, which threatened to cost them their careers. So, in order to lose the weight again, the young models became bulimic or began to use amphetamines or cocaine. "In Paris, every model I met took cocaine," Bean said. Yet, if a model's usage of drugs becomes known, photographers will no longer hire her. "Good photographers won't touch a model who is into drugs." A drug habit quickly begins to show in the model's eyes and nostrils and that can cost the photographer money.

These days, many models start their careers at fourteen, fifteen, or sixteen. The fashion industry demands youth. Yet at these young ages, teenagers don't know how to deal with the realities of a competitive business in which they may be finished before they're twenty. Journalist Marcelle Clements researched what happens to these young models and concluded that "the worst victims are the ones who . . . become 'stars'—as stardom is thought of in the fashion business."[6] They come to New York, primarily, and quickly earn what seems like a huge sum of money. They're pampered, painted, petted. Soon they begin to believe, because they have today's "look," that they're above having to behave professionally.

One fashion editor told Clements, "I can't stand having to work with these little girls who've done one cover and think they're stars. Oh, of course, I do it if we're dying to have that face. And I put up with all the crap they pull at the shooting. Going into the bathroom to snort. Throwing tantrums. I'll put up with anything to get a good session. But it drives me crazy when they behave unprofessionally. They think they're stars, and they forget—or never understood—that this is a business."

It's hard, however, for a fifteen-year-old to have that kind of maturity. Few do, and because of that, they burn out early. As a successful makeup artist said, after a short while in the business, the very young models tend to "get that tough, bitchy look." That can't be fixed with makeup. When they no longer look fresh, innocent, young, their careers end as quickly as they began.

Even more mature, professional models who manage to stay away from the lures of drugs and bizarre diets can become seduced by their own images. Former top model Erin Grey, now an actress, says, "When you face a mirror all day long and you look at yourself and analyze yourself and manicure yourself and you're constantly dealing with your image, after a while, your sense of who you are is, 'I am my hair, my face, my makeup.' It takes you over whether you realize it or not. This habitual process becomes a form of identification—this thing you create."[7]

A successful model might begin to believe that her only value is her beauty. If it fades, she ceases to exist. Also, like the rest of us, models get older, and few of the older high fashion models remain employed. Erin Grey recalls, "When you're twenty-eight years old and you're told that you're too old, it's pretty shocking. It's shocking when you've been at the top of your career and you're used to a six-figure income, and suddenly you've got to start all over again."

Most fashion models don't work in the business once they're past thirty. The industry demands youth. As a result, the picture that's presented to us over and over again—the picture we try to match—is that of youthful beauty.

Commercial models last longer than fashion models. A commercial model, who may also be an actress, does television commercials or print ads in which she's supposed to look like what agent Jeannette Walton calls "real people." A successful commercial model, Walton says, "projects personality as much as beauty. In this business, the requirement is the ability to project a happy, satisfied, successful personality. 'Look at me, look how happy and successful I am because I eat cornflakes,' " is what the model in a cereal ad tries to convey to the reader or viewer. Because a commercial model represents the so-called average consumer, there is more leeway in her appearance. She might be the business executive selecting an insurance policy. She might be the housewife with a headache swallowing a couple of aspirin. She might be the friendly-looking grandmother talking on the telephone to her grandchildren.

Yet even with commercial models, beauty is important. They may be slightly shorter and heavier than high fashion models, but they are more attractive than a cross section of the general public. They are usually not fat; they don't have many visible wrinkles; they haven't got crooked teeth or noses; their hair is always perfectly arranged. The woman executive in an ad will not wear her hair in a bun and wire-rimmed glasses on her nose; she'll be prettier than most of our friends. That housewife with a headache will look better than most of us do on days when we feel our best. Television's idea of a grandmother might look fifty-five, but she'll seldom look seventy. Of their "type," each of these women will be extremely good-looking. They are so conspicuous that we think of them as our norm.

Yet clearly these models are not representative of the general public, starting with their age. Researchers Paula England, Alice Kuhn, and Teresa Gardner examined advertisements in five national magazines over a twenty-year period.[8] "Though only 27 percent of U.S. adult women are under thirty," they found, "77 percent of the women portrayed in ads appeared under thirty. Only 4 percent of the women in the ads were judged to be forty or over, despite the fact that 57 percent of adult women are at least forty."

The media present an inaccurate picture of women. The ideal represented in the magazines, on television, on the movie screen, is almost invariably younger and more beautiful than average, and younger and more beautiful than we are. By observing the media, as well as by succumbing to various societal pressures, we learn to feel insecure about our own looks—increasingly so as we age.

One model who's trying to break the anti-aging tradition of the advertising industry and the media is Kaylan Pickford, who is gray-haired and in her fifties. Tall and slender, Pickford has the body of a woman twenty years younger. On the other hand, her fine-boned, beautiful face, with its strikingly blue eyes, is the face of a middle-aged woman. Her look is quite sophisticated, but it's middle-aged sophisticated.

Pickford began her modeling career when she was forty-five years old. Recently widowed, she was searching for a career in which she would meet people and earn money. It was not an easy search. "I was a mid-life woman with no resume," she says. "It's very rough in this society because none of the things you become very good at as a homemaker apply most of the time [to paid jobs]."

An agent noticed Pickford and convinced her that she should try modeling. She had some success, but soon branched into acting in television commercials to increase her income. She rails at being hired mainly for what she calls "the repair kit" ads, the ones for denture cleaners, laxatives, headache remedies, hemorrhoid cures. "That's what you get a call to go to work for if you're a middle-aged woman."

Pickford is very outspoken about how television twists our perceptions of older women. "We live in a culture that for twenty-five solid years [since television became a fixture in the typical home] has sold us one image, which is youth, and I think that has had a terrible backlash on everybody. The media as much by omission as commission have said [older women] don't exist . . . that we're not viable sexually [because] we're not young. We see endless pictures of the older man and the very young woman. What does that say? It says that the older man is acceptable and the older woman isn't. She's missing. It's saying at the same time that an older woman cannot be beautiful, cannot be sexual."

Pickford feels that advertisers are being terribly shortsighted not to recognize the market that middle-aged and older women comprise. "There's not a single fashion store in [New York] today that uses anyone my age in their *catalogs*," she claims. "And yet it is women my age who are spending the money. *I* am their shopper and nobody is appealing to me.

"I do not yet see any ads, either in print or commercials that show a woman [like me] in fashions, driving a car, smoking a cigarette, having a drink, wearing perfume, anything. They are not using models [my age] in these ads. Look at the soft drink ads. Who do they think is drinking all those sugar-free diet sodas? And yet there's not one person my age in them."

Los Angeles Times television critic Howard Rosenberg agrees with Pickford that advertisers misrepresent and devalue older women. With slight exaggeration, he says, "When you have a long-running detergent commercial implying that the hands of the average thirty-year-old woman are spotted and gnarled, you're selling a powerful bias [against aging women], not just detergent."[9]

There's a lot of money to be made in convincing us that our natural aging process is repulsive. Currently, for example, many skin care products aim their advertising and sales campaigns at women who fear getting older. In a commercial for one such product, classically beautiful actress Catherine Deneuve peers from the television screen, saying, "Take a closer look. This year I'll be forty . . . I've got nothing to hide." The product Deneuve is hyping, Youth Garde, is backed by a multimillion-dollar advertising and promotion budget.

There are no estimates of the total dollar amount that all manufacturers together spend on such advertising because companies have differing methods of calculating their ad budgets and many keep such expenses secret. But, as an example, *Advertising Age,* the industry's Bible, estimated that Oil of Olay spent more than $26 million on advertising in 1982.

Model Kaylan Pickford believes that advertising's youth bias is actually detrimental to young people as well as to older people. Youth "begin to think they have something special, that they're *it,* that they have to accomplish everything they need to accomplish by the time they are thirty. That's a setup for failure, making it an emotionally devastating thing to reach the age of thirty."

Pickford speculates that her presence on the TV screen and occasionally in a magazine gives the false impression that advertising opportunities are opening up for middle-aged models. However, the backbone of most models' careers is catalog work, for which she is not hired. "I don't work every day. Financially is the only way I can judge this. Financially, I'm a long way behind a young top model. My hourly rate is not less, it's the same, but it's a question of supply and demand . . . and if there's no demand for your age, you can't work."

Pickford does note some changes, however. The fact that she works *at all* is progress. She also published a book, *Always a Woman,* in 1982, which couples photographs of herself with her philosophy about aging as an American woman. Five years earlier, when she began writing, "nobody would talk to me about the book." The media decided that no one would be interested in reading about a middle-aged woman and her ideas about life and beauty. Recently, however, Pickford was approached by a Hollywood producer who is considering filming a television movie of her life.

Beauty and youth are also of great importance for women in another media profession that has profound influence in this country, that of television journalist. Advertisers have been quick to pick up on this fact. Television commercial actress Nina Mann says, "There are lots of calls for a Mary Tyler Moore type [in commercials]. Female reporters have become the role models for women of intelligence and ability."[10]

According to Los Angeles psychologist Anita Siegman, a full 80 percent of her college-age female clients who suffer from bulimia aspire to become TV news anchors. In her opinion, for young women from upper middle class, conservative families, being on television in a news capacity is considered more respectable than working as an actress or model. Yet the result, media exposure and possible stardom, is the same.

Barbara Matusow, author of *The Evening Stars: The Rise of the Network News Anchor,* says that in virtually every city in the country, "the news is delivered by an anchor 'team': a cast of characters carefully designed to represent a kind of 'pseudo-family' with which viewers can identify. Indeed, news consultants often hear people tell them how much better they like a certain anchor team than they do their own families. These TV families tend to follow a certain pattern: All have a father figure, and perhaps a sassy younger brother or sister. But the role of mother is largely absent."[11]

The role of "sister" in this TV family is most often played by a woman who is not only young (or at least appears to be young) but is very attractive as well. Although many within the news business insist that it's journalistic talent and not appearance that counts for female reporters and anchors, it's rare that a homely woman is seen on the air. Even with pretty newscasters, station management is likely to try to improve their looks. For instance, when Judy Woodruff became a news anchor in Atlanta a decade ago, she was told to cut her long hair. In 1979, Mary Alice Williams was urged by NBC's New York station to change her eye color by wearing tinted contact lenses. In 1980, Dorothy Reed was forbidden by ABC's San Francisco station to braid her hair in corn rows.[12]

A double standard concerning appearance has existed since the first woman was hired to appear in front of the camera. The queen of television news reporters, Pauline Frederick, who was NBC's United Nations correspondent for twenty-two years, recalls her first major television assignment, covering the national political conventions in 1948. Even in those early days, Frederick was advised that her appearance was important. "I went to Elizabeth Arden to learn about makeup and to Bonwit Teller to learn about how to dress [for television], and always I got plenty of advice on how I should look. Management wanted me in navy colors with austere necklines. They insisted I lighten my dark brown hair. They told me to wear contact lenses instead of glasses. And they continually had my hair teased because they said I was too flat-headed."

Throughout her long career, Frederick realized that "when a man got up to speak, people listened, then they looked, then they continued to listen. When a woman got up to speak, first they looked, and then if they liked what they saw, they listened."[13]

Other prominent women television journalists like Frederick have been outspoken about the importance of their looks. Liz Trotta of CBS, who is in her mid-forties, told *TV Guide,* "I've been in television since 1965 and I'm an expert on this—not on anything else, but on this—and I can tell you that anybody who says that a woman's looks aren't the number one factor is just whistling 'Dixie'! Her reporting ability is definitely number two. A woman is still supposed to look pert and upbeat, not like Edward R. Murrow. People still say to me—constantly—'Don't look so serious on the tube, Liz. Show those teeth! Use that charm!' And whenever they put a woman on the nightly news, they're going to say it's because she's an excellent journalist who just happens to look like Sophia Loren."[14]

It's reasonable that any broadcaster, female or male, should seem pleasant and intelligent. Noticeable physical defects and deformities might well distract from what is being communicated. But "pleasant and intelligent" allows far more variation in appearance than most stations do. It's true that a few forward-looking stations are deviating from the "thin youthful beauty" norm for female television reporters. WABC-TV in New York City features not only ample-sized Phyllis Eliasberg as its consumer reporter, but gray-haired Katie Kelly as its film critic. Ruth Ashton Taylor, who is in her fifties and admits to having had cosmetic facial surgery, has been an on-camera reporter at Los Angeles's KNXT-TV for many years. Nevertheless, these women are exceptions. More frequently, a woman who doesn't fit the television news ideal simply doesn't work in front of the camera.

Perhaps the most visible example of this is the case of Christine Craft, who in 1983 won a half-million-dollar judgment against Metromedia, the former owner of Kansas City station KMBC. (A judge later overturned Craft's victory and the case was retried in January, 1984. In the retrial, a Federal jury in Joplin, Missouri, awarded Craft $325,000. As of this writing, Metromedia was expected to appeal this decision.) Craft claimed that KMBC's management had dropped her as an anchorwoman in 1981 because she was "too old, unattractive and not deferential enough to men."[15]

Christine Craft, a former schoolteacher, began her television career when she was thirty—a rather late start for such an appearance-conscious business. She worked at stations in Salinas and San Francisco, California, and later was hired as a weekend reporter for a segment of "CBS Sports Spectacular" in New York. It was in this job that she first ran up against TV's emphasis on beauty for women. The program managers had her naturally brown hair bleached platinum, her eyebrows dyed black, and her mouth painted into a beestung look. Craft didn't like it.

When she interviewed for the anchor position at WMBC in 1980, she says she told the station management about her experience with "Sports Spectacular" and that she resented being "made over." She didn't want that to happen again and felt that, if WMBC didn't like the way she looked, "they should not have hired me."

But they did hire her and, soon after, they began to try to change Craft's appearance. She says that KMBC news director Ridge Shannon "said I was a good reporter, but they [the station's management] were always insulting me about the way I look. My face wasn't symmetrical; my hair was too messy. I tried to block it out." Craft also said that she was constantly being compared with a female anchor at a competing station, a twenty-three-year-old former model who did not function as a reporter in the field, as Craft herself sometimes did.

According to Craft, a talent consultant "drew a railroad track down the side of my face, white circles around each eye—like a panda in reverse. I was a good sport. I let them pile this crap on my face, even though I felt like someone in Kabuki makeup." KMBC's next step was to hire a fashion consultant to select Craft's wardrobe and give her a chart directing which clothes she was to wear on camera each day.

Despite all these efforts to change her, in August, 1981, Craft was informed that Kansas City residents—especially women in the twenty-six-to-thirty-nine age group that advertisers seek—found her to be "too old, unattractive and not deferential enough to men." She would be allowed to work out her contract as a reporter, but she was finished as an anchorwoman.

Craft refused to be demoted. She later commented to TV critic Howard Rosenberg, "If I was so terrible looking that people had to turn their dials, then this wasn't the place for me. Can you imagine how I felt? I didn't like to be thought of as an ugly old hag."

Craft, an attractive woman now in her late thirties, surmises that she surprised KMBC's management when she not only didn't leave quietly, but filed suit. "They never expected a woman to admit she was told she was unattractive. You know how vain we're supposed to be. But they decided to play hard ball with the wrong person."

Until recently, television could claim that there were few if any older women reporting the news simply because women hadn't been in the business long enough to grow older. Now, however, television may be at a crossroads. Barbara Walters is over fifty and she's still on the air. Other prominent women network journalists are either already over forty or fast approaching that watershed age. Still, the fact is that they all look younger than they are. Marlene Sanders states that "if I didn't, I wouldn't be on the air, despite my credentials, which are twenty-five years' worth of everything!"[16]

It remains to be seen whether these women, as their wrinkles and creases begin to show through their makeup, will experience the same type of discrimination that Kaylan Pickford finds in modeling. In the meantime, one kind of role model predominates in television news: an unusually young and pretty woman. And, because the TV journalist displays her brains as well as her beauty, she is even more intimidating to female viewers than are actresses and models. She offers a difficult standard to meet.

Most of us don't aspire to being on the cover of *Vogue* or extolling the virtues of an advertiser's floor wax or even explaining the day's news to television viewers. Yet that doesn't stop us from wanting to be as appealing as these women are. Or to be more precise, to be as appealing as we *think* they are. That daughter figure on the evening newscast is not only beautiful and intelligent, but seems respected and happy as well. She belongs to a "family" which has been carefully constructed to appeal to us as viewers.

Commercials and advertisements are even more carefully constructed to create a longing in the consumer. For example, let's consider an advertisement in which a beautiful young model dressed in fashionable evening clothes and jewelry is being helped into an expensive car by a handsome, distinguished-looking man. This ad is supposed to make us desire the automobile. However, we're being sold more than a car. We're also being sold the idea that, if we resembled this model, we, too, would be wealthy enough to dress the way she does, attract a man like hers, and be as happy as she is.

We should not forget what a big business advertising is. We can get a fair idea of the size of the ad business by comparing some *Advertising Age* statistics.[17] This newspaper first reported billing figures for the largest advertising agencies back in 1945, when the twenty-two biggest agencies billed a total of $515 million dollars. In comparison, *Advertising Age* reported that in 1981 the largest agency in America, Young & Rubicam, billed $2.35 billion, four times as much as the top twenty-two agencies in 1945. The billings for the top twenty-two agencies in 1981 totalled nearly $24 billion.

With such phenomenal sums at stake, it's not surprising that advertising continues to sell us an image of youthful beauty and affluence. We spend billions of dollars for products and services in the attempt to "buy" ourselves a life-style akin to the one in that automobile ad. As long as we fail to achieve that life-style, we're likely to keep on spending money in a futile attempt to realize that dream.

Ads for beauty products are even more direct in selling us that glamorous image than are ads for other commodities. Beauty product ads imply that, with the right eye shadow or face cream or lipstick, we'll be as exciting, successful, sexy, and happy as the models wearing them in the photographs. There's plenty of evidence that we believe it. The cosmetics and toiletries industry in America, for instance, is a multibillion-dollar business. The retail value of skin care products alone, according to the Department of Commerce, was $2.5 billion in 1981. Retail sales of fragrances were estimated at nearly $2 billion in the same year, and those of hair preparations at more than $2 billion.

Profits for the cosmetics industry have been rising about 10 percent annually since the mid-seventies, despite the economy's battles with inflation and recession.[18] The highest sales of cosmetics are charted in the South, followed by the West, the Northeast, and the Midwest, in descending order. The naked face of the late sixties and early seventies is no longer fashionable.

Wearing makeup can be fun, of course. Most people agree that when it's tastefully applied, makeup improves our appearance. When we think we look good, chances are that we exude more self-confidence and actually become more attractive to others in a number of ways.

But making up our faces also allows us to feel that we can mask ourselves when we meet the world, that we can create a persona different from our real selves. Susan Sontag has said that "a woman's face is the canvas upon which she paints a revised portrait of herself. One of the rules of this creation is that the face *not* show what she doesn't want it to show. Her face is an emblem, an icon, a flag. How she arranges her hair, the type of makeup she uses, the quality of her complexion—all these are signs, not of what she is 'really' like, but of how she asks to be treated by others, especially men."[19]

Yet, if we do not conform to the current norm of wearing makeup, others may perceive us negatively, as though we didn't care enough about ourselves or about them to take the trouble. These perceptions can be particularly important on the job. For instance, studies done by Jean Ann Graham, Ph.D., a social psychologist in the dermatology department of the University of Pennsylvania, found that a woman wearing makeup is more likely to be considered outgoing, confident, and competent than if she wore none.[20]

A study conducted in Britain for an American cosmetic company documented the fact that many working women wore cosmetics on the job because they felt that it was expected of them or that cosmetics helped them to present a "better image."[21]

The way in which we make up our faces can serve as an emblem of social status, too, just like the kind of clothing we wear. Garish or overdone makeup labels a woman from a lower-class background, while understated makeup marks her as being from a higher stratum of society. Wearing no makeup at all, at least in the eighties, may be interpreted as meaning that the woman is lazy, unfashionable, or making a political statement. No matter what we do about makeup, people judge us by it.

Perhaps the least desirable effect of facial cosmetics is the dependency they might foster in us. I know a woman who declares with pride that she has never allowed her husband to see her without her false eyelashes. She feels that this attention to makeup proves that she loves him. After all, she goes to a lot of trouble to ensure that he sees her only when she is at her best. Yet I wonder what she is afraid he would see in her unadorned face? She is symbolically masking her real self from the person with whom she should feel most able to be honest and free. Los Angeles psychotherapist Laura Schlessinger reminds us that "if you want to be loved for yourself, you've got to show yourself. It's true that when you fix yourself up nice, you're showing self-respect, self-regard. You're willing to take the time to be well groomed. But when that becomes an inordinately powerful focus in your life, you've become distorted and won't be happy."

Unfortunately, it seems that many of us have become convinced that without our makeup, our masks, we are unfit for others to see. We must recognize an important distinction. In a healthy sense, using makeup demonstrates that we respect ourselves, but feeling that we are repulsive *without* the aid of artifice shows only self-loathing. Along the same lines, there is a big difference between wearing a dash of perfume because we think that it adds to our allure and believing that *without* the perfume, our natural odor is repulsive. The first is evidence of a healthy self-image, the second self-hatred. Yet, in either case, the behavior we exhibit to others is quite the same.

Unfortunately, that British study revealed a surprising amount of basic self-loathing among women who relied on cosmetics. The researchers reported, "The retention of youthfulness was of great concern to those interviewed and many women revealed an enormous dependency on cosmetics, never allowing themselves to be seen without cosmetics. Some were trying to conceal specific defects while others seemed to feel *they did not exist* without cosmetics." When these women were asked for a one-word description of how they felt without makeup, they replied with such adjectives as: "ghastly," "lifeless," "dowdy," "terrible," and "frumpy."

The researchers reported a much heavier reliance on makeup among women who did not work and were therefore dependent upon their husbands for status. It was essential to them to look beautiful to their husbands without appearing to use many cosmetics. As a result, like the woman with the false eyelashes, many of the British women conducted their beauty routines secretly. From a third to a half of the women surveyed were convinced that, without cosmetics, their sex appeal would dwindle.

With these kinds of attitudes, it's easy to understand why some of us actually believe that our lives will change if we switch our lipstick, our hair color, our face cream. Lives don't change because of such products, of course. Yet instead of realizing the invalidity of our beliefs, we tell ourselves that we just haven't found the right product yet. Maybe the next lipstick will do the trick, perform the magic, transform us into someone we are not.

We often harbor such expectations of hairdressers, too. Successful hairdressing schools today teach students not only how to style hair, but also some elementary psychology. Hairdressers need it, because so many women bring their problems with them to the beauty shop, expecting them to be solved by a new permanent wave or hair color.

Beverly Hills stylist Tracy Hill, who has styled hair and trained other hairdressers for more than two decades, describes this phenomenon. For women who are insecure, she says, going to the beauty salon can be "like plastic surgery. They think they're going to become a different personality. They want to come in five four and go out five seven and thin just because of their hair."

One of Hill's longtime clients is a good illustration. After twenty years of marriage, the woman discovered that her husband was having an affair. "She had her hair color changed, she had a perm, she had her hair cut differently. She had it all done and the husband left her anyway. But, in her mind," changing her hairdo would solve the problems in her life.

Hill adds that many women bring in a photograph of a movie star or model and ask to have their hairstyle copied.

"They believe that there's magic in looking like a star, that some of the star's magic will rub off on them if they look like her." Most women will choose an actress or model who looks vaguely like them. Perhaps they have a similar nose or smile or hair color. Seldom will they ask to look like a totally different type. For instance, "very seldom will a blonde bring in a picture of Liz Taylor."

Our unrealistic hopes about a hairdresser's ability may well be a reason that so many of us find them intimidating. New York assertiveness trainer Perla Knie says that women in her workshops view hairdressers as authority figures, like doctors and lawyers. She admits that she once put up with a haughty hairstylist because he kept telling her, "If it wasn't for me, you'd still look like Brooklyn."[22] Like many women, Knie wanted to believe that her hairdresser had "some secret, magical knowledge that would make me look right."

Since looking "right" is so important to our self-image, our very identity, we dare not offend someone who can remove our inherent flaws and help us achieve this ideal. We sometimes give our hairdressers an absurd amount of power because we believe they have the capability to solve our problems, simply by making us more beautiful.

The truth is that our appearance almost never is that intimately related to our problems.

It's important that we be realistic. What we see on television, in the movies, in the magazines, in the catalogs is not reality. It's nothing more than a fantasy carefully constructed to sell us goods and services. As a by-product, we are being sold an erroneous norm for women in our society.

There's nothing wrong with purchasing goods and services, of course. Yet, if we purchase an automobile not because we need one but because we hope to resemble the beautiful woman in the advertisement, we may be disappointed with our purchase. A new lipstick will not transform us into a happier person. A visit to the beauty parlor will not entice a wandering husband back home.

We must weed out the fantasy from the reality. We must refuse to allow the media to make us feel inadequate because we don't match the image of ideal beauty they show us. Our value is not based on whether or not we look like a fashion model or a television journalist or a famous actress. It's based upon our own unique combination of personality and intelligence, spiced with our individual looks.

As model Kaylan Pickford puts it, "The essential thing is to become independent in your thinking, not to be swayed, to realize that you're being brainwashed. If it's making you feel bad about yourself as a female, turn off that damned machine, and don't read the magazines!"

We may buy the products the media sell us, but we should not buy the concept that we must be young and beautiful to be worthwhile as human beings.

12

ESCAPING THE BEAUTY TRAP

The first step in escaping from the beauty trap is simply to realize that it exists and to admit to ourselves that we have become trapped. We must acknowledge that we have overblown expectations of physical attractiveness, and we must admit that chasing elusive and transient feminine beauty is a loser's game. Only then can we begin to change our self-image and move toward self-love.

As we have seen, we are bombarded from every side throughout our lives with the message that a woman *is* her appearance. It starts in infancy, when we are first valued for our prettiness. Our attractiveness soon becomes an essential element in forming sexual identity. Our beauty (or lack of it) affects our family relationships, our friendships, our academic careers. Society constantly tries to sell us products and services by reiterating that beautiful is best—and that beauty can be purchased. Under this kind of pressure, it's hard not to believe that physical beauty is the most important asset in a woman's life. It's hard not to swallow the concept that with beauty, a woman will have everything and that, without it, she will have nothing.

Yet we must realize that these beliefs are inherently self-destructive. Adhering to them robs us of time, money, energy, and self-esteem. Beauty cannot deliver the power it promises.

Because beauty's sole purpose is to attract others, its power is secondhand at best, of a weak and transient variety. By concentrating our efforts on pursuing beauty, we risk failure to achieve real power, economic freedom, and self-reliance. We risk never achieving the life that taking overt action will gain for us. Also, because none of us is capable of physical perfection for long, we risk setting ourselves up for constant failure.

The second step in freeing ourselves from the beauty trap is making a decision that we do, in fact, *want* to escape. Some women don't, of course. They find more rewards in staying where they are, although those rewards ultimately are negative. For example, some women may be comfortable with the essential passivity of pursuing beauty. It's certainly easier not to take risks. It's easier to attach unrealistic expectations to having breasts enlarged or losing twenty pounds or changing a hair color than it is to try actively to realize dreams and desires.

Remaining in the beauty trap also allows us to wallow in self-pity, which for some is reward enough.

It allows us to postpone our lives indefinitely, too. As soon as we lose weight (or can afford the right wardrobe, or have a face-lift, or clear up acne), we can tell ourselves, *then* we'll change jobs (or get married, or go back to school, or make new friends.) It's easy to hinge any life change that we claim to want, yet really are afraid to make, on a future change in physical appearance. Again, we give ourselves an excuse for passivity.

Staying in the beauty trap also provides a handy target for an unending list of personal problems. If a husband leaves, for instance, it's easier to believe he left because his wife was unattractive rather than because she was uncommunicative. If others are promoted over us at work, it's easier to believe we were passed over because we've got a few facial wrinkles than because our efforts are not up to par. It's easier to target our lack of social relationships on overweight than it is to change our personalities. We assume less responsibility for a lack of beauty than for personal failures.

Remaining in the beauty trap also has the advantage of conformity. Most women, after all, are still caught there. Staying there allows us to commiserate, to wallow in a sort of group self-pity. We can sit around and reassure each other that we're all in the same sinking boat, enjoying a certain sense of doomsday camaraderie.

The last reason for staying in the beauty trap may well be the hardest for us to admit, atonement for the guilt of achieving "unfeminine" power. As I researched this book, I met many outgoing women, some who held top-level jobs, others who were highly educated and proud of their achievements. Yet they felt that they had somehow failed as women because they were not beautiful enough. Some of these women have become as compulsively hardworking about beautifying themselves as they are about their careers. They spend their lunch hours exercising, their vacations at fat farms, their money on "miracle cures" for the aging process.

Power does not conform to the feminine stereotype or the ideal of womanhood that our society has taught us we *should* fit. Therefore, according to this stereotype, a woman who has real power in the world must be unfeminine. If, somewhere deep inside ourselves, we believe this, despite wanting and seeking our own power, we are in emotional conflict. A typical way of resolving this conflict is to become even more "feminine" in another stereotypical way, to become more beautiful. Or at least to attempt it. Perhaps many powerful women feel that, by being even more beautiful than the traditionally passive and dependent woman, they will no longer be labeled unfeminine. Or, perhaps, they will no longer *feel* unfeminine.

Unfortunately, physical beauty is not necessarily achieved artificially, at least not indefinitely. Even highly accomplished women are doomed to eventual failure if they remain in the beauty trap.

Escaping the beauty trap does not mean that we must give up caring about and enhancing our appearance. The free woman enjoys the heady feeling of looking her best and noticing others' admiring glances as much as anyone else. Still, she has physical beauty in the proper focus.

If we are to take the third step and emerge from the beauty trap, we must alter our system of beliefs about femininity and physical appearance. With the help of the many experts I interviewed for this book, I've compiled the following suggestions to make that task easier for all of us.

Recognize that a woman's looks do not determine her worth. This ingrained belief can be combated if we examine it carefully. What I found helpful was to make a list of women I truly admire and then determine why. Almost none of the women on my list were physically beautiful by strict popular standards. They included a few famous women like Eleanor Roosevelt and Lillian Hellman, as well as a variety of my friends and acquaintances. To me, they were beautiful in quite a different way—who they were, not what they looked like, determined their attractiveness. Once I recognized that I didn't even admire the Playmate of the Month, my perspective on beauty began to change.

Acknowledge traits in yourself that you admire and develop new ones. Again, a list can be helpful. My own list included such qualities as perseverance, creativity, and intelligence. A friend's personal list added kindness and humor. When your list is complete, compare it with the traits possessed by your most admired women. Chances are you share several admirable qualities with them.

Now look at those traits that you don't share with your most admired women but would like to, such as a sense of humor or empathy for other people. By redirecting your time and energy toward developing these qualities and skills in yourself, your self-image will surely improve. With increased self-love, you will begin to exhibit another, more lasting kind of beauty, inner beauty.

Other people will recognize this beauty in you, too. Studies at Hofstra University have shown that an average-looking woman who is warm and considerate will be considered good-looking by other people.[1] Similarly, Hanover College psychologist Roger L. Terry has determined that facial *expression* is more important than any single feature in determining beauty. Certainly facial expression is a reflection of our attitudes, toward ourselves as well as toward others.

Discuss the beauty trap with other women. This helps us realize that we are not alone. One of my most valuable insights in writing this book was to recognize that the beauty trap is so encompassing. When I discussed the book's concept with other women, many expressed immediate recognition, saying with relief, "I thought *I* was the only one who felt that way." Talking about these feelings openly helps destroy the beauty trap's power over us.

Discuss the importance of physical beauty with your man. Ask your husband or lover or friend what qualities he most values in you, and chances are, your appearance will be far down on his list. For many men, intelligence, compassion, wit, and other assets outshine the importance of physical attractiveness.

In addition, we tend to become blind to most flaws in people we love, particularly physical imperfections. Does your man's slight paunch make you love him less? Are you ready to leave him if he goes bald? If not, why should you fear his leaving you because of your appearance? If you express your concerns to him, you'll probably receive valuable reassurance in return. If you don't, the relationship might be doomed anyway.

The biggest risk of the beauty trap in a loving relationship is that we concentrate our efforts on beauty to the detriment of other, more substantial and lasting qualities.

Learn to appreciate your beauty instead of dwelling on your flaws. If you can't think of any physically beautiful asset you possess, ask your friends, your family, your lover. Every woman is beautiful in some way, whether she has lovely skin, or legs, or hair, or breasts, or eyes. A friend of mine who was feeling depressed decided to write down every compliment she received over a week's time. Normally, her habit was to concentrate only on negative remarks. By compiling a list, she forced herself to remember the compliments, and, at the end of the week, she was happily surprised to realize how many times people had expressed appreciation of her.

We might apply the same system to beauty. If someone says, "Your hair looks nice today," write it down. If you receive a compliment on your dress, write it down. In time, you will begin to see yourself in a new light and to recognize assets that might be enhanced.

Eventually, if you *feel* more beautiful, others will actually begin to perceive you that way. Pennsylvania State University's Dr. Richard Lerner conducted an experiment in which he determined that the more attractive a woman *thought* herself to be, regardless of her actual appearance, the more beautiful she seemed to others.[2] For these women, he said, "beauty was in the eyes of the beholdee."

Set aside a specific amount of time for beauty rituals. A woman who is thoroughly caught in the beauty trap may spend many hours each day primping, exercising, shopping for clothes, even simply worrying about her looks. If we don't notice these hours slipping by, we soon learn that there's little time left over for developing other aspects of ourselves or for pursuing other interests.

Each of us should budget whatever amount of time she chooses, as long as she sticks to her schedule. I decided that I would allow myself enough time to swim several mornings a week, which helps me reduce tension as well as control my weight. Then I give myself an additional twenty minutes a day for my hair and makeup. Except for special occasions, I feel I can't afford to spend any more time than that. Practically, this limits my hairstyle and the elaborateness of my makeup routine.

Another woman might choose to spend either more or less time than I do, of course. The idea is to acknowledge how much time we are spending on self-beautification and to limit that time.

Budget the money spent on beauty as carefully as the time. For one woman, such a budget might include many thousands of dollars for extensive plastic surgery; for another, it might be limited to a few dollars for inexpensive makeup. The key point is to stop spending both impulsively and compulsively because beauty cannot be purchased. We need to recognize just how much money we spend on beauty-related products and services and to be sure that we're spending thoughtfully.

A woman who used to be a "clothes horse" finally realized that she was nearly bankrupting herself buying clothes she could not afford. She made out a realistic clothing budget, then limited her purchases. As a result, she altered her buying habits, concentrating on classic styles instead of fads. In a year's time, she had not only paid off all her charge accounts, she had begun accumulating a small art collection with her savings. Because of her new spending priorities, she's feeling more satisfied with herself.

Vow not to perpetuate the beauty trap. For those of us who have daughters, this is a particularly important point. The attitude that keeps women prisoners of their self-image has been passed down from mothers to daughters. We can help our daughters escape this legacy by showing them how society lures females into the beauty trap and by helping them learn to value themselves far more than their physical appearance.

In addition, all of us, whether we have daughters or not, can help to destroy the beauty trap by passing on our new-found knowledge of its dangers to all women—our friends, our sisters, our own mothers. Finally, we should stop judging other women by their appearance.

Remaining in the beauty trap results in a lifelong downward spiral of depression and self-loathing. However, we can change historical predecent and free ourselves. Attracting a man with our physical beauty is no longer our only method of survival, or our only means of personal happiness or professional success.

By achieving our own personal power, we can begin to bargain in the world with a new kind of currency. When we begin to value ourselves because we offer more lasting qualities than physical beauty, so will others.

In the final analysis, it's the woman who sees far beyond her own mirror who is most attractive to herself and to everyone around her. It's the woman who has a sure sense of her own value who attracts others to her.

When Socrates said, "Beauty is a short-lived reign," he meant physical beauty. Inner beauty—the only true beauty—is not transient. It lasts a lifetime.

Thus, only by freeing ourselves from the beauty trap, only by creating our own new definition of beauty, can we become and remain truly beautiful.

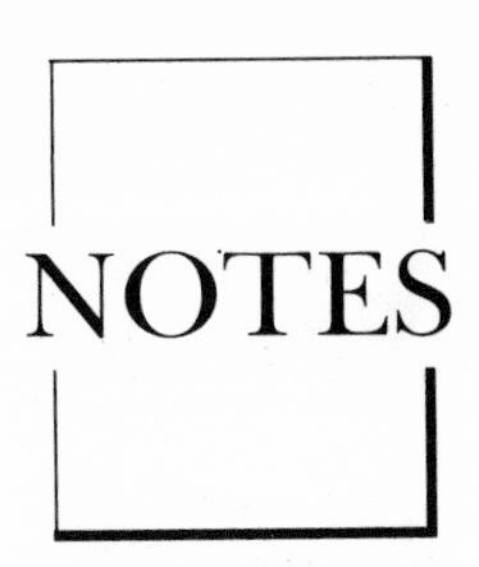

NOTES

CHAPTER 2

1. This letter was reprinted in *The Undercover Story,* a 1982 publication of the Fashion Institute of Technology.

CHAPTER 3

1. See "Survey on Body Image, Weight, and Diet of College Students," by Toby Mark Miller, R.D., Judith Gilbride Coffman, R.D., and Ruth A. Linke, Ph.D., which was published in the *Journal of the American Dietetic Association* for November, 1980.
2. This survey, "Women: What's on Their Minds? What's in Their Hearts? What Do They Fear? What Do They Hope For?" appeared in the January, 1983, issue of *Glamour.*
3. This survey was cited in "Worry Scale: What We Fear Most and Least," in *American Health* for September/October, 1983.
4. Lena Horne's comments on beauty were included in "My Mother Lena Comes from a Line of Proud Women," by Gail Lumet, published in the August, 1981, issue of *Ms.*
5. Princess Grace's remarks were recalled in a *Los Angeles Times* obituary, "Princess Grace Dies of Injuries After Car Crash," by Jack Jones. It appeared in the September 15, 1982, edition.
6. Candice Bergen was quoted in "Interview: Bergen and Bisset—The Beauty and the Beauty," in *Vogue* for August, 1981.
7. Jodie Foster was quoted in Bob Colacello's article "Why Jodie Foster Won't Quit," in the December 11, 1983, issue of *Family Weekly.*
8. Sandy Duncan's comments were included in "Ask Them Yourself," in the August 13, 1983, issue of *Family Weekly.*

9. Dr. Theodore Isaac Rubin's remarks in this chapter are quoted from his "Psychiatrist's Notebook" column in *Ladies' Home Journal* for May, 1981.
10. The Mathews study and the University of Illinois study mentioned in the following paragraph are cited in the article "Beauty Can't Be Beat," by Glenn Wilson and David Nias, which appeared in *Psychology Today* for September, 1976.
11. Alice Walker wrote about her childhood injury in "When the Other Dancer Is the Self," which appeared in *Ms.* for May, 1983.
12. Jessica Lange was quoted in Cyndi Stivers's article "Jessica Lange: From Frog to Movie Princess," which appeared in *Life* for March, 1983.
13. Diane Sawyer was the subject of "CBS's New Morning Star," by Harry Waters, which appeared in *Time* for March 14, 1983.
14. Jane Fonda's dieting problems were cited in "5 Bodies to Die For and How They Got That Way," in *Glamour* for January, 1983.
15. Goldie Hawn mentioned her teen-age self-image problems to Barbara Walters on ABC-TV during the week of July 25, 1983.
16. Debra Winger's remarks were taken from Chris Chase's article "Debra Winger in Terms of Success," which appeared in *The New York Times* on December 4, 1983.
17. Anjelica Huston was quoted by Roderick Mann in his article "She's Grown Accustomed to Her Face," which appeared in the *Los Angeles Times* on April 14, 1983.
18. Christina Ferrare was quoted in Sherry Suib Cohen's article "The Million Dollar Models," which appeared in *Ladies' Home Journal* for August, 1982.
19. Debbie Reynolds's comments were included in "Woman of the Year: Debbie Reynolds," by Andrea Chambers, which appeared in the March 14, 1983, issue of *People.*
20. Maya Angelou was quoted by Paul Rosenfield in his article "Angelou: The Caged Bird Still Sings," in the *Los Angeles Times* on May 29, 1983.

CHAPTER 4

1. Sherry Black Kozloff and other attractive, successful women in business discussed their experiences in an article by Elizabeth Wheeler, "The Perils of Pretty," in the May, 1981, issue of *Working Woman.*
2. Ellen Berscheid was interviewed on "America's Obsession with Beautiful People" in *U.S. News & World Report,* January 11, 1982.
3. Beneke, Timothy. *Men on Rape.* New York: St. Martin's Press, 1982.
4. This segment of the "Toni Grant Show" was aired on ABC radio on July 18, 1983.
5. Madeline E. Heilman has written about her research in two publications: "Sometimes Beauty Can Be Beastly," *The New York Times,* June 22, 1980; and with co-researcher Lois R. Saruwatari in "When Beauty is Beastly: The Effects of Appearance and Sex on Evaluations of Job Applicants For

Managerial and Nonmanagerial Jobs," *Organizational Behavior and Human Performance,* 1979.

6. Florence W. Kaslow and Lita L. Schwartz published the results of their study in "Self-Perceptions of the Attractive, Successful Female Professional," *Intellect Magazine,* February, 1978.
7. A report about the Bar-Tal and Saxe study, "Beauty Makes the Beast Look Better," appeared in *Psychology Today* in August, 1976. Bar-Tal and Saxe published their study in the June, 1976, issue of *Personality and Social Psychology.*

CHAPTER 5

1. This study, "The Eye of the Beholder: Parents' Views on Sex of Newborns," by J. Z. Rubin, J. J. Provenzano, and Z. Luria, appeared in the *American Journal of Orthopsychiatry,* Vol. 44, 1974.
2. Susan Williams's letter to the editor appeared in the July 30, 1983, edition of the *Los Angeles Times.*
3. Letty Cottin Pogrebin wrote about parents' preference for sons in her book *Growing Up Free,* published by McGraw-Hill in 1980. Other comments of Pogrebin's in this chapter are also from *Growing Up Free.*
4. Dr. Alice Baumgartner's survey appeared in the February, 1983, issue of *Redbook* and was also the subject of Ann Landers's syndicated newspaper column for May 17, 1983.
5. Dr. Ross D. Parke's comments on his research appear in his book *Fathers,* published by Harvard University Press in 1981.
6. Elena Gianini Belotti's book *What Are Little Girls Made Of?* analyzes the roots of feminine stereotypes. It was published in the United States by Schocken Books in 1976.
7. Signe Hammer's book *Passionate Attachments: Fathers and Daughters in America Today* was published by Rawson Associates in 1982.
8. *The Psychology of Sex Differences,* by Eleanor Emmons Maccoby and Carol Nagy Jacklin, was published by Stanford University Press in 1974.
9. *Father Power,* by Henry Biller, Ph.D., and Dennis Meredith, is a 1974 publication of David McKay Company.
10. Karen Rowe was quoted in Charles Solomon's article "Was Snow White a Snow Job?" which appeared in the *Los Angeles Times* on July 16, 1983.
11. Bill Barton's comment was quoted in the October 18, 1983, issue of the Rochester (New York) *Times Union.*
12. Dr. Sam Janus was quoted by Beverly Beyette in her article "Are Children Losing Their Childhood?" which appeared in the *Los Angeles Times* on September 2, 1981.
13. This study and others are discussed by Ellen Berscheid and Elaine Walster in their article "Beauty and the Best," which was published in *Psychology Today* in March, 1972.

14. Karen Dion's findings are summarized in her article "Physical Attractiveness and Evaluation of Children's Transgressions," *Journal of Personality and Social Psychology,* Vol. 25, No. 2, 1972.
15. "Reactions to a Child's Mistakes as Affected by Her/His Looks and Speech," by Leonard Berkowitz and Ann Frodi, was published in *Social Psychology Quarterly,* Vol. 42, No. 4, 1979.
16. Richard Lerner's comments appeared in "Personality Molds Your Looks—So Think Attractiveness," by Richard Wolkomir, *Science Digest,* February, 1979.
17. Mary Vespa wrote about children's beauty contests in "A Two-Year-Old in False Eyelashes," *Ms.,* September, 1976.

CHAPTER 6

1. Dr. Dabbs's comments appeared in "Teen Suicide," by Mary Susan Miller, *Ladies' Home Journal,* February, 1977.
2. Maccoby and Jacklin's comments are taken from their book *The Psychology of Sex Differences.*
3. Natalie Shainess's study, "A Re-evaluation of Some Aspects of Femininity Through a Study of Menstruation: A Preliminary Report," appears in *Science and Psychoanalysis,* Vol. 5, edited by Jules H. Masserman, M.D., and published by Grune & Stratton in 1962.
4. Signe Hammer's book *Daughters and Mothers, Mothers and Daughters* was published by Quadrangle/The New York Times Book Co., in 1976.
5. Dr. Biller's comments, like those in the previous chapter, are taken from his book *Father Power.*
6. Professor Sanford M. Dornbusch discussed his research on the influence that peer groups have on children at the Southern California Stanford Conference, held in Los Angeles, March 2, 1980.
7. Carin Rubinstein, Phillip Shaver, and Letitia Anne Peplau are authors of "Loneliness," an article published in the February, 1979, issue of *Human Nature.*
8. Drs. Daniel Offer, Eric Ostrov, and Kenneth I. Howard are authors of *The Adolescent, a Psychological Self-Portrait,* which is based on their study. The book was published in 1981 by Basic Books.
9. The figures in this and the following paragraph are taken from the Alan Guttmacher Institute's report *Teen Pregnancy: The Problem that Won't Go Away,* published in 1981.

CHAPTER 7

1. Berscheid and Walster reported the results of their computer dance in their article "Beauty and the Best," which appeared in the March, 1972, issue of *Psychology Today.*

2. Helen Gahagan Douglas's comments about Eleanor Roosevelt originated in *The Eleanor Roosevelt We Remember,* 1963, and were reprinted in Elaine Partnow's book *The Quotable Woman,* published by Pinnacle Books in 1980.
3. Carol Burnett was quoted in Phyllis Battelle's article, "Carol Burnett: 'There's Something Different About Me,' " which appeared in *Ladies' Home Journal* for August, 1983.
4. Trudi Ferguson was quoted in Barbara Baird's article, "Women Cite 'Femininity' in Success," which appeared in the *Los Angeles Times* on November 10, 1983.
5. These figures were released by the Census Bureau in 1980.
6. "100 Men Tell What They Love About Women" appeared in *Glamour* for April, 1983.
7. Schvaneveldt and Cannon's study was mentioned in "Weighing Traits of Prospective Mates," which appeared in *Family Weekly* for March 26, 1983.
8. Dr. Joyce Brothers's remarks appear in her book *What Every Woman Should Know About Men,* published in 1982.
9. Dr. Pietropinto's remarks are taken from the book he coauthored with Jacqueline Simenauer, *Beyond the Male Myth.* It was published in 1977 by New American Library.
10. Berscheid and Walster discussed these studies in their *Psychology Today* article. See note 1.
11. Alan Feingold reported his findings in "Testing Equity as an Explanation for Romantic Couples 'Mismatched' on Physical Attractiveness," which appeared in *Psychological Reports,* Vol. 49, 1981, pp. 247–250.
12. Carol Thurston's findings received national press coverage and also were the subject of her article "Deliberation of Pulp Romances," in the April 1983 issue of *Psychology Today.*
13. See Chapter 4 for a further discussion of Madeline Heilman's research on the effect of physical appearance in the workplace.
14. Mary Cunningham aired her anger in an article that she wrote for the July, 1981, issue of *Working Woman,* "Mary Cunningham on Corporate Ethics and Sexual Prejudice."
15. Ellen Goodman's comments appeared both in her nationally syndicated newspaper column and in Jane Adams's article about Mary Cunningham and Jane Pfeiffer, "Fallen Idols," which appeared in the February, 1981, issue of *Working Woman.*
16. These statistics are from The Continental Group Report, 1983.
17. Statistics released by the Census Bureau in 1980 indicated that the U.S. divorce rate had increased 96 percent since 1970.

CHAPTER 8

1. Berscheid's study is noted in her article with Elaine Walster, "Beauty and the Best," *Psychology Today,* March, 1972, and also in Glenn Wilson and

David Nias's article, "Beauty Can't Be Beat," *Psychology Today,* September, 1976.

2. Jack Lemmon was quoted in Jerry Cohen's article "Jack Lemmon: 'I Think I Have a Lot of Kid in Me,'" which appeared in the *Los Angeles Times* on May 3, 1983.
3. Kathleen Fury's article, "Clash or Smash? Would the Legendary Beauty and the Great Comic Hit It Off?" appeared in the September 3, 1983, issue of *TV Guide.*
4. Susan Sontag's essay, "The Double Standard of Aging," appeared in the September 23, 1972, issue of *Saturday Review.*
5. Patty Moore was profiled in "Old Before Her Time," by Katherine Barrett, which appeared in *Ladies' Home Journal* for August, 1983.
6. Dyan Cannon's remarks were quoted in Bart Mills' article, "Dyan Cannon, Nonagenarian," which appeared in the February 5, 1984, *Los Angeles Times.*
7. Dr. Rita Ransohoff made these and other remarks as main speaker on a panel titled "Venus After Forty," at the fourth annual Women in Crisis conference, held in New York City, in November, 1982.
8. Lance Morrow wrote "In Praise of Older Women," for the April 24, 1978, issue of *Time.*
9. "Staying Fit and Fantastic at Any Age," written by Eric Levin and reported by David Wallace, appeared in the April 11, 1983, issue of *People.*
10. Doris Jonas Freed was quoted by Beverly Stephen in her article "Prenuptials: Taking No Chance on Love," which appeared in the February 17, 1983, *Los Angeles Times.*
11. Maggie Scarf's book on female depression, *Unfinished Business: Pressure Points in the Lives of Women,* was published in 1980 by Doubleday.
12. This survey was reported in the September, 1983, issue of *Weight Watchers* magazine and also by United Press International early that same month.

CHAPTER 9

1. This statistic is from NBC News "Monitor," aired on June 11, 1983.
2. The Virginia Slims Poll is cited in "Body Image," by Carol Lynn Mithers in *Mademoiselle,* July, 1980.
3. The *Glamour* magazine survey was illustrated by InfoGraphics and distributed to newspapers. It appeared in the Santa Monica *Evening Outlook* on January 5, 1983.
4. The Metropolitan Life Insurance statistics appeared in "Who's Setting the Thin Trend?" by Julie Hatfield, which appeared in the *Boston Globe* on October 14, 1982.
5. "Cultural Expectations of Thinness in Women," by David M. Garner, Paul E. Garfinkel, Donald Schwartz, and Michael Thompson, appeared in *Psychological Reports,* Vol. 47, 1980.

6. Dr. Margaret Mackenzie was quoted by Muriel Dobbin in her article "Dieting to 'Get Control' Over Our Lives," which appeared in the *Los Angeles Times* for August 27, 1982.
7. Dr. Baila Zeitz is quoted in "How Dieting Can Affect Your Job," by Linda Heller, which appeared in the April, 1983, issue of *Working Woman.*
8. Dr. Charles Lucas was quoted in "Life After the Loss of Weight," by Judy Klemesrud, which appeared in the October 12, 1982, edition of *The New York Times.*
9. These numbers were computed by using the Metropolitan Life Insurance Company's weight chart, as published in *Newsweek* on March 14, 1983.
10. Dr. Reubin Andres was quoted by Steve Franzmeier in his article "National Quest for Average American Full of Surprises," which appeared in the *Los Angeles Times* on December 9, 1983.
11. This study of Canadian girls and their eating habits was published in the March, 1983, issue of the *Journal of the American Dietetic Association* and was also reported by United Press International.
12. Fifteen-year-old Julie Merson's comments appeared in her letter to the editor of the *Los Angeles Times* on April 23, 1983.
13. Dr. Preston Zucker's comments appear in the foreword to *Treating and Overcoming Anorexia Nervosa,* by Steven Levenkron, M.D., published in 1982 by Charles Scribner's Sons.
14. Dr. Raymond E. Vath, who treated Cherry Boone O'Neill, wrote a chapter in her book *Starving for Attention,* which was published by Continuum in 1982. His comments are quoted from that chapter.
15. Dr. Steven Levenkron's quotes are from his book *Treating and Overcoming Anorexia Nervosa.* See note 13.
16. Leslie Gershman was quoted in "A Deadly Feast and Famine," in *Newsweek* for March 7, 1983.
17. Cherry Boone O'Neill's story is told in greater detail in her book *Starving for Attention.* See note 14.
18. Dr. Joel Yaeger's comment was quoted by Joan Sweeney in "A Cultural Paradox—Food Abuse," which appeared in the *Los Angeles Times* on July 18, 1983.
19. This UCLA study was mentioned in "Clinical Programs Offer Help to Bulimics," by Rose Dosti, which appeared in the *Los Angeles Times* on February 24, 1983.
20. The response to the British television program was noted in Jane Brody's article "An Eating Disorder of Binges and Purges Reported Widespread," which appeared in *The New York Times* on October 20, 1981.
21. The University of Minnesota study is mentioned in Joan Sweeney's article. See note 18.
22. Dr. Fima Lifshitz's study was mentioned in a United Press International story published in the Santa Monica *Evening Outlook* on September 1, 1983; the study was also the subject of an article Dr. Lifshitz co-wrote for the

September 1, 1983, issue of *The New England Journal of Medicine.* Co-authors of "Fear of Obesity: A Cause of Short Stature and Delayed Puberty" are M.T. Pugliese, G. Grad, P. Fort, and M. Marks-Katz.

23. Dr. Katherine A. Halmi's research was noted by Joan Sweeney in her *Los Angeles Times* article. See note 18.
24. Suzanne Gordon's remarks are quoted from her editorial "The Balanchine Look Starves the Women of Ballet," which appeared in the *Los Angeles Times* on July 18, 1983.
25. Kim Chernin's quotes in this paragraph and the following are taken from her article "How Women's Diets Reflect Fear of Power," which appeared in *The New York Times* on October 11, 1981.

CHAPTER 10

1. Information about Ann-Margret's accident and her quotes are taken from three articles: "Ann-Margret—Fate Hasn't Been Kind but She's Still Fighting Back," by Sheila Weller, which appeared in *Ladies' Home Journal* for November, 1978; "Overworked and Overwrought, Ann-Margret Wants to Become the Girl Who Can Say 'No!' " by Cutler Durkee, which appeared in *People* for December 18, 1978; and "The Price of Being Ann-Margret," by Paul Rosenfield, which appeared in the February 13, 1983, edition of the *Los Angeles Times Calendar.*
2. UPI health editor Patricia McCormack's report on Jacqueline Auriol appeared in the August 20, 1982, edition of the *Los Angeles Times.*
3. Betty Rollin's book *First You Cry* was published by J. B. Lippincott in 1976.
4. Sandra Pesmen quotes Dr. Brenda Solomon in her article "Is There Life After a Mastectomy?" which appeared in the February 5, 1978, issue of the *Los Angeles Times.*
5. See "After Mastectomy: Choosing to Look Different," by Paula Armel in *MS.* for July, 1981.
6. Lucia Greene Connolly wrote about Patty Fischer's experience in "A New Drug for Cystic Acne Gives Patty Fischer's Face and Spirit a Lift," for *People,* June 27, 1983.
7. Betty Ford was quoted in "The Unveiling of a New Ford," which appeared in the October 23, 1978, edition of *Time.*
8. Carol Burnett was quoted in "With a Long-Postponed Trip to the Dentist, Carol Burnett Lets Her Beauty Bloom," by Eleanor Hoover. The article appeared in *People* for July 4, 1983.
9. Mariel Hemingway was quoted by Roderick Mann in "The 'Other' Hemingway, Star of 'Star,' " which appeared in the *Los Angeles Times* on November 8, 1983.
10. Dr. Molnar was quoted in "Cosmetic Surgery: A Risky Route to Youth, Beauty?" by Orr Kelly, Abigail Trafford, and Joanne Davidson. It appeared in *U. S. News & World Report* for August 9, 1982.

11. Dr. Grossman was quoted in Diana Benzaia's article "Your First Face-Lift: What Can Go Wrong," which appeared in *Harper's Bazaar* for September, 1982.
12. Dr. Strahan's comments are taken from "Cosmetic Surgery: A Risky Route to Youth, Beauty?" See note 10.
13. Dr. Robert Spence was quoted by Gerri Kobren in her article "Surgical Removal of Fat Formations Not Without Risk," which appeared in the February 27, 1983, issue of the *Los Angeles Times.*
14. Irma Shorell's remarks were taken from Mary Rourke's article, "Avoiding the Drawbacks to Plastic Surgery," which appeared in the September 23, 1983, *Los Angeles Times.*

CHAPTER 11

1. Ellen Berscheid was quoted in "America's Obsession With Beautiful People," which appeared in *U. S. News & World Report,* January 11, 1982.
2. Nina Blanchard was quoted by Michael Capaldi in his article "Tough Advice to Starry-Eyed Street Kids," which appeared in the *Los Angeles Times* on February 2, 1983.
3. Christie Brinkley's earnings were mentioned in "The Packaging of Christie Brinkley," by Mark Goodman, which appeared in the March 13, 1983, issue of *Family Weekly.*
4. The average earnings of a New York model were reported in Julie Hatfield's article, "The Darker Side of Modeling," which appeared in the *Boston Globe* on March 3, 1983.
5. Linda Bean's quotes are taken from Julie Hatfield's article. See Chapter 9, note 4.
6. Marcelle Clements's article, "The Model Game," appeared in *Mademoiselle* for July, 1983.
7. Erin Grey's comments were taken from Kenneth R. Clark's article "Ex-Model Lives High-Fashion Past in TV Movie," which appeared in the Santa Monica *Evening Outlook* for October 30–31, 1982.
8. "The Ages of Men and Women in Magazine Advertisements," by Paula England, Alice Kuhn, and Teresa Gardner appeared in the Autumn, 1981, issue of *Journalism Quarterly.* The national magazines examined included *Vogue, Ladies' Home Journal, Ms., Playboy,* and *Time,* for the years from 1960 to 1979. This research project was funded by a grant from the National Institute of Mental Health.
9. Howard Rosenberg's comment was taken from his article "TV Sells Youth Image, Elderly Pay the Price," which appeared in the December 10, 1982, issue of the *Los Angeles Times.*
10. Nina Mann was quoted by Linda Bird Francke in "Advertising Grows Up," which appeared in *Newsweek,* March 19, 1979.
11. Barbara Matusow's remarks are taken from an editorial she wrote for the

August 14, 1983, *Los Angeles Times,* "TV News Anchor-Families: There's No Room for Mom."

12. The experiences of these three TV journalists were reported by William A. Henry III in "Requiem for TV's Gender Gap?" which appeared in *Time* for August 22, 1983.
13. Pauline Frederick's quotes were taken from Clarke Taylor's article "The Perils of Pauline Frederick," which appeared in the September 24, 1983, issue of the *Los Angeles Times,* and from Philip Nobile's article, "TV News and the Older Woman," which appeared in *New York* for August 10, 1981.
14. Liz Trotta was quoted by Joan Barthel in her article "Power to the Women," which appeared in *TV Guide* on August 13, 1983.
15. Christine Craft's quotes were taken from a series of articles written by TV critic Howard Rosenberg. They appeared in the *Los Angeles Times* between April 12, 1982, and August 10, 1983.
16. Marlene Sanders was quoted in "Power to the Women." See note 14.
17. These figures appear in the March 24, 1982, issue of *Advertising Age.*
18. These statistics on the growth of the cosmetics industry are taken from Jan Hoffman's article "Making Up Is Hard to Do," which appeared in the *Village Voice* for May 31, 1983.
19. This quote is from Susan Sontag's essay "The Double Standard of Aging," which appeared in *Saturday Review* on September 22, 1972.
20. Jean Ann Graham's findings were cited in "What's Wrong with a Bare Face?" which appeared in the April, 1983, issue of *Glamour.*
21. This survey and others are reported in *The Cosmetic Benefit Study,* conducted from January through August, 1978, by Project Associates, Inc., and published by the Cosmetic, Toiletry and Fragrance Association, Inc.
22. Perla Knie was quoted by Georgia Dullea in her article "Standing Up to the Hairdresser Can Take a Kind of Courage," which appeared in the January 12, 1981, issue of *The New York Times.*

CHAPTER 12

1. The studies done at Hofstra University and by Dr. Roger L. Terry are noted in Richard Wolkomir's article, "Personality Molds Your Looks—So Think Attractiveness," which appeared in *Science Digest* for February, 1979.
2. Dr. Richard Lerner's studies were noted in Richard Wolkomir's *Science Digest* article. See note 1.

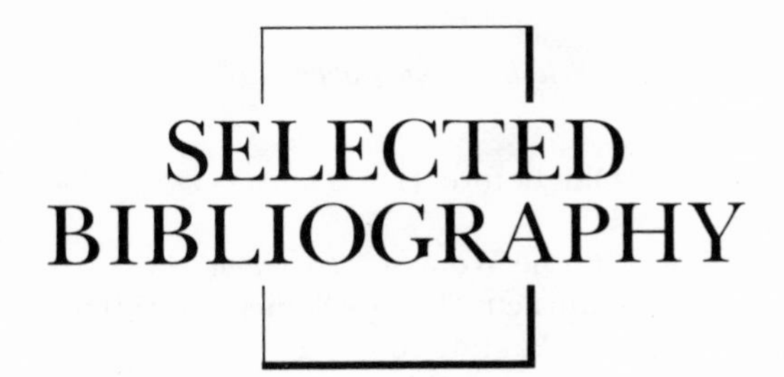

SELECTED BIBLIOGRAPHY

Abbott, Aaron A., and Sebastian, Richard J. "Physical Attractiveness and Expectations of Success." *Personality and Social Psychology Bulletin,* September, 1981.

Adams, Gerald R. "Social Psychology of Beauty: Effects of Age, Height and Weight on Self-Reported Personality Traits and Social Behavior." *Journal of Social Psychology,* December, 1980.

Adams, Jane. "Fallen Idols: Was 1980 a Bad Year for Women." *Working Woman,* February, 1981.

Adler, Jerry, and Gosnell, Mariana. "What It Means to Be Fat." *Newsweek,* December 13, 1982.

"America's Obsession with Beautiful People." *U. S. News & World Report,* January 11, 1982.

"Anorexia Nervosa: A Brain Shrinker?" *Science News,* October 23, 1982.

"Anorexia Nervosa: An Eating Disorder." *Current Health,* September, 1981.

Armel, Paula. "Choosing to Look Different." *Ms.,* July, 1981.

"Ask Them Yourself." *Family Weekly,* August, 1983.

Baker, Nancy C. "If You're Always Eating on the Job, It May Not Be Because You're Hungry." *Working Mother,* March, 1982.

———. "A New Kind of Breast Surgery: Norma Hertzog's Victory Over Cancer." *Good Housekeeping,* August, 1983.

———. *New Lives for Former Wives: Displaced Homemakers.* New York: Anchor Press/Doubleday, 1980.

———. "Why Women Stay with Men Who Beat Them." *Glamour,* August, 1983.

Bardwick, Judith M. *Psychology of Women.* New York: Harper and Row, 1971.

Barrett, Katherine. "Old Before Her Time." *Ladies' Home Journal,* August, 1983.

Barthel, Joan. "Power to the Women." *TV Guide,* August 13, 1983.

Battelle, Phyllis. "Carol Burnett: 'There's Something Different About Me.'" *Ladies' Home Journal,* August, 1983.

Beck, Kay. "Television and the Older Woman." *Television Quarterly,* Summer, 1978.

Belotti, Elena Gianini. *What Are Little Girls Made Of? The Roots of Feminine Stereotypes.* New York: Schocken Books, 1976.

Beneke, Timothy. *Men on Rape: What They Have to Say About Sexual Violence.* New York: St. Martin's Press, 1982.

Benzaia, Diana. "Your First Face-Lift: What Can Go Wrong." *Harper's Bazaar,* September, 1982.

Berkowitz, Leonard, and Frodi, Ann. "Reactions to a Child's Mistakes as Affected by Her/His Looks and Speech." *Social Psychology Quarterly,* Vol. 42, No. 4, December, 1979.

Berscheid, Ellen, and Walster, Elaine. "Beauty and the Best." *Psychology Today,* March, 1972.

Biller, Henry, and Meredith, Dennis. *Father Power.* New York: David McKay Co. 1974.

Blakely, Mary Kay. "Youth and Beauty, Age and Wisdom." *Vogue,* November, 1981.

Bolotin, Susan. "Voices from the Post-Feminist Generation." *New York Times Magazine,* October 17, 1982.

Bonnett, Margie. "If You Think Beautiful People Hold All the Cards, You're Right, Says a Researcher." *People,* July 7, 1980.

Bridges, Judith S. "Sex-Typed May Be Beautiful, but Androgynous Is Good." *Psychological Reports,* February, 1981.

Bridgwater, Carol Austin. "Bad News About Looking Too Good." *Mademoiselle,* May, 1981.

Brothers, Joyce. *What Every Woman Should Know About Men.* New York: Simon & Schuster, 1982.

Burns, Cherie. "An Insider's View of Beauty Pageants." *Seventeen,* September, 1980.

Bush, Sherida. "Beauty Makes the Beast Look Better." *Psychology Today,* August, 1976.

"The Business of Being Beautiful." *Harper's Bazaar,* January, 1979.

Calvert, Catherine. "Body Image." *Mademoiselle,* July, 1980.

Chambers, Andrea. "Woman of the Year: Debbie Reynolds." *People,* March 14, 1983.

"The Changing Face of the American Beauty." *McCall's,* April, 1976.

"Chemistry of Beauty: Makeup as Medicine." *Science Digest,* August, 1982.

Chernin, Kim. "How Women's Diets Reflect Fear of Power." *The New York Times Magazine,* October 11, 1981.

———. *The Obsession: Reflections on the Tyranny of Slenderness.* New York: Harper & Row, 1981.

Clements, Marcelle. "The Model Game." *Mademoiselle,* July, 1983.

Cohen, Sherry Suib. "The Million Dollar Models." *Ladies' Home Journal,* August, 1982.

Connolly, Lucia Greene. "A New Drug for Cystic Acne Gives Patty Fischer's Face and Spirit a Lift." *People,* June 27, 1983.

Corliss, Richard. "The New Ideal of Beauty." *Time,* August 30, 1982.

Cunningham, Mary. "Mary Cunningham on Corporate Ethics and Sexual Prejudice." *Working Woman,* July, 1981.

Devol-VanLieu, Shirley. "Psychosocial Adaptation to Postmastectomy Reconstructive Mammoplasty." Unpublished doctoral dissertation for the University of Southern California, 1981.

Dion, Karen. "Physical Attractiveness and Evaluation of Children's Transgressions." *Journal of Personality and Social Psychology,* Vol. 25, No. 2, 1972.

Dowling, Colette. *The Cinderella Complex: Women's Hidden Fear of Independence.* New York: Summit Books, 1981.

Durkee, Cutler. "Overworked and Overwrought, Ann-Margret Wants to Become the Girl Who Can Say 'No!' " *People,* December 18, 1978.

England, Paula; Kuhn, Alice; and Gardner, Teresa. "The Ages of Men and Women in Magazine Advertisements." *Journalism Quarterly,* Autumn, 1981.

Feingold, Alan. "Testing Equity as an Explanation for Romantic Couples 'Mismatched' on Physical Attractiveness." *Psychological Reports,* Vol. 49, August, 1981, pp. 247–250.

Fishel, Elizabeth. *Sisters: Love and Rivalry Inside the Family and Beyond.* New York: Wm. Morrow & Co., 1979.

"5 Bodies to Die For and How They Got that Way." *Glamour,* January, 1983.

Francke, Linda Bird, and Whitman, Lisa. "Advertising Grows Up." *Newsweek,* March 19, 1979.

Friday, Nancy. *My Mother, My Self.* New York: Delacorte Press, 1977.

Friedan, Betty. *The Feminine Mystique.* New York: Dell Publishing, 1963.

———. *The Second Stage.* New York: Summit Books, 1981.

Fury, Kathleen. "Clash or Smash? Would the Legendary Beauty and the Great Comic Hit It Off?" *TV Guide,* September 3, 1983.

Garner, David M.; Garfinkel, Paul E.; Schwartz, Donald; and Thompson, Michael. "Cultural Expectations of Thinness in Women." *Psychological Reports,* Vol. 47, October, 1981.

Geise, L. Ann. "The Female Role in Middle Class Women's Magazines from 1955–1976: A Content Analysis of Nonfiction Selections." *Sex Roles,* Vol. 5, No. 1, 1979.

Gesell, Arnold, M.D.; Ilg, Frances L., M.D.; and Ames, Louise Bates, Ph.D. *The Child from Five to Ten.* New York: Harper & Row, 1977.

Goldberg, Phillip A.; Gottesdiener, Marc; and Abramson, Paul R. "Another Put-Down of Women? Perceived Attractiveness as a Function of Support for the Feminist Movement." *Journal of Personality and Social Psychology,* Vol. 32, No. 1, 1975.

Goodman, Mark. "The Packaging of Christie Brinkley." *Family Weekly,* March 13, 1983.

Gordon, Suzanne. *Off Balance: The Real World of the Ballet.* New York: Pantheon, 1983.

Gottlieb, Paula Gribetz. "My Side: Betty Friedan." *Working Woman,* February, 1982.

Greer, Germaine. *The Female Eunuch.* New York: McGraw-Hill Book Co., 1970.

"Growing Old, Feeling Young." *Newsweek,* November 1, 1982.

Halas, Celia, and Matteson, Roberta. *I've Done So Well—Why Do I Feel So Bad?* New York: Ballantine Books, 1978.

Halcomb, Ruth. "Do Pretty Women Get Ahead?" *Mademoiselle,* October, 1981.

Hammer, Signe. *Daughters and Mothers, Mothers and Daughters.* Quadrangle/The New York Times Book Co., 1975.

———. *Passionate Attachments: Fathers and Daughters in America Today.* New York: Rawson Associates, 1982.

Harris, Janet. *The Prime of Ms. America.* New York: G. P. Putnam's Sons, 1975.

Haskell, Deborah. "The Depiction of Women in Leading Roles in Prime Time Television." *Journal of Broadcasting,* Spring, 1979.

Heilman, Madeline E., and Saruwatari, Lois R. "When Beauty is Beastly: The Effects of Appearance and Sex on Evaluations of Job Applicants for Managerial and Non-Managerial Jobs." *Organizational Behavior and Human Performance,* 1979.

Heilman, Madeline E., and Stopeck, Melanie H. "Being Attractive, Advantage or Disadvantage? Performance Based Evaluations and Recommended Personnel Actions as a Function of Appearance, Sex and Job Type." Unpublished paper for New York University, 1983.

Heller, Linda. "How Dieting Can Affect Your Job." *Working Woman,* April, 1983.

Hennig, Margaret, and Jardim, Anne. *The Managerial Woman.* New York: Pocket Books, 1976.

Henry, William A., III. "Requiem for TV's Gender Gap?" *Time,* August 22, 1983.

Holahan, Carole Kovalic, and Stephan, Cookie White. "When Beauty Isn't Talent: The Influence of Physical Attractiveness, Attitudes Toward Women and Competence on Impression Formation." *Sex Roles,* August, 1981.

Hoover, Eleanor. "With a Long-Postponed Trip to the Dentist, Carol Burnett Lets Her Beauty Bloom." *People,* July 4, 1983.

Horn, Jack. "Beauty Does as Beauty Is: How Looks Influence Liking." *Psychology Today,* August, 1974.

Howard, Jane. *A Different Woman.* New York: E. P. Dutton & Co., 1973.

Howe, Louise Kapp. *Pink Collar Workers.* New York: Avon Books, 1977.

Ilg, Frances L., M.D.; Ames, Louise Bates; and Baker, Sidney, M.D. *Child Behavior: Specific Advice on Problems of Child Behavior.* New York: Harper & Row, 1981.

"Interview: Bergen and Bisset—The Beauty and the Beauty." *Vogue,* August, 1981.

Jamison, Kay R.; Wellisch, David K.; and Pasnau, Robert O., M.D. "Psychosocial Aspects of Mastectomy: II. The Man's Perspective." *American Journal of Psychiatry,* May, 1978.

———. "Psychosocial Aspects of Mastectomy: I. The Woman's Perspective." *American Journal of Psychiatry,* April, 1978.

Jarvis, Jeff. "Reveling in the Lap of Luxury." *People,* March 21, 1983.

Kanekar, Suresh, and Kolsawalla, Maharukh B. "Responsibility of a Rape Victim in Relation to Her Respectability, Attractiveness and Provocativeness." *Journal of Social Psychology,* October, 1980.

Kanner, Bernice. "She Brings Home the Bacon and Cooks It: Madison Avenue Thinks They'll Keep Her." *Ms.,* March, 1980.

Kelly, Orr; Trafford, Abigail; and Davidson, Joanne. "Cosmetic Surgery: A Risky Route to Youth, Beauty?" *U. S. News & World Report,* August 9, 1982.

Kaplan, Helen Singer, M.D. *The New Sex Therapy: Active Treatment of Sexual Dysfunctions.* New York: New York Times Book Co., 1974.

Kaslow, Florence W., and Schwartz, Lita L. "Self-Perceptions of the Attractive, Successful Female Professional." *Intellect Magazine,* February, 1978.

Kleiger, Estelle. "Vanity in the 19th Century." *American History,* August, 1979.

Levenkron, Steven. *Treating and Overcoming Anorexia Nervosa.* New York: Charles Scribner's Sons, 1982.

Levin, Eric, and Wallace, David. "Staying Fit and Fantastic at Any Age." *People,* April 11, 1983.

Levine, Suzanne, and Lyons, Harriet, eds. *The Decade of Women: A Ms. History of the Seventies in Words and Pictures.* New York: Paragon Books, 1980.

Light, Leah L.; Hollander, Steven; and Kayra-Stuart, Fortunee. "Why Attractive People are Harder to Remember." *Personality and Social Psychology Bulletin,* June, 1981.

Linedecker, Clifford L. *Children in Chains: An Angry Look at the Shame of*

Our Nation—Sexual Exploitation of the Young. New York: Everest House, 1981.

Lips, Hilary M., and Colwill, Nina Lee. *The Psychology of Sex Differences.* Englewood Cliffs, N. J.: Prentice-Hall, 1978.

Lumet, Gail. "My Mother Lena Comes from a Line of Proud Women." *MS.*, August, 1981.

Maccoby, Eleanor Emmons, and Jacklin, Carol Nagy. *The Psychology of Sex Differences.* Stanford, Ca.: Stanford University Press, 1974.

Masserman, Jules H., M.D., ed. *Science and Psychoanalysis,* Vol. 5. New York: Grune & Stratton, 1962.

Matusow, Barbara. *The Evening Stars: The Rise of the Network News Anchor.* New York: Houghton Mifflin, 1983.

Mayer, Anne. "The Gorge-Purge Syndrome." *Health,* July, 1982.

McCoy, Kathleen. *Coping with Teenage Depression.* New York: New American Library, 1982.

Miller, Mary Susan. "Teen Suicide." *Ladies' Home Journal,* February, 1977.

Miller, Toby Mark; Coffman, Judith Gilbride; and Linke, Ruth A. "A Survey on Body Image, Weight, and Diet of College Students." *Journal of the American Dietetic Association,* November, 1980.

Mithers, Carol Lynn. "Body Blindness." *Mademoiselle,* May, 1983.

———. "I Wasn't Always Pretty." *Mademoiselle,* June, 1982.

Morgan, Robin. *Sisterhood Is Powerful: An Anthology of Writings from the Women's Liberation Movement.* New York: Random House, 1970.

Morrow, Lance. "In Praise of Older Women." *Time,* April 24, 1978.

"1983 Women's Views Study." *Glamour,* January, 1983.

Nirenberg, Sue. "Life Without Father." *Savvy,* March, 1983.

Nobile, Philip. "TV News and the Older Woman." *New York,* August 10, 1981.

Offer, Daniel; Ostrov, Eric; and Howard, Kenneth I. *The Adolescent, A Psychological Self-Portrait.* New York: Basic Books, 1981.

Olds, Ruthanne. *Big and Beautiful: Overcoming Fatphobia.* Washington, D.C.: Acropolis Books, 1982.

"100 Men Tell What They Love About Women." *Glamour,* April, 1983.

"100 Years of Good Looks." *McCall's,* April, 1976.

O'Neill, Cherry Boone. *Starving for Attention.* New York: Continuum, 1982.

Parke, Ross D. *Fathers.* Cambridge: Harvard University Press, 1981.

Partnow, Elaine. *The Quotable Woman.* Los Angeles: Pinnacle Books, 1980.

Pecoraro, Tom. "Jurors Go Easy on Handsome Rapists with Homely Victims." *Psychology Today,* October, 1981.

Pennebaker, James W. "Truckin' with Country-Western Psychology." *Psychology Today,* November, 1979.

Penney, Alexandra. "Seduction by Packaging." *The New York Times Magazine,* November 18, 1979.

Peterson, John L., and Miller, Constance. "Physical Attractiveness and Marriage Adjustment in Older American Couples." *Journal of Psychology*, July, 1980.

Pickford, Kaylan. *Always a Woman.* New York: Bantam Books, 1982.

Pietropinto, Anthony, M.D., and Simenauer, Jacqueline. *Beyond the Male Myth.* New York: New American Library, 1977.

Pogrebin, Letty Cottin. *Growing Up Free: Raising Your Child in the 80's.* New York: Bantam Books, 1981.

Powell, Barbara. *How to Raise a Successful Daughter.* Chicago: Nelson-Hall, 1979.

Project Associates, Inc. *The Cosmetic Benefit Study.* Washington, D.C.: The Cosmetic, Toiletry and Fragrance Association, Inc.

Rich, Adrienne. *Of Woman Born: Motherhood as Experience and Institution.* New York: W. W. Norton & Co., 1976.

Roiphe, Anne. "Exteriors." *California Living,* January 16, 1983.

Rollin, Betty. *First You Cry.* Philadelphia: J. B. Lippincott Co., 1976.

Rubenstein, Carin. "The Diet Doubters." *Psychology Today,* August, 1982.

———. "Sex Repel." *Psychology Today,* December, 1979.

Rubenstein, Carin; Shaver, Phillip; and Peplau, Letitia Anne. "Loneliness." *Human Nature,* February, 1979.

Rubin, J. Z.; Provenzano, J. J.; and Luria, Z. "The Eye of the Beholder: Parents' Views on Sex of Newborns." *American Journal of Orthopsychiatry,* Vol. 44, 1974.

Rubin, Theodore Isaac, M.D. "Putting Looks in Perspective." *Ladies' Home Journal,* May, 1981.

Scarf, Maggie. *Unfinished Business: Pressure Points in the Lives of Women.* New York: Doubleday, 1980.

Seligman, Jean. "A Deadly Feast and Famine." *Newsweek,* March 7, 1983.

———. "Keep Your Double Chins Up." *Newsweek,* March 14, 1983.

"Sexual Aesthetics." *Science Digest,* August, 1982.

Shaw, Bill. "Before She Beat Anorexia—Pat Boone's Daughter Cherry Nearly Starved to Death." *People,* October 11, 1982.

Sontag, Susan. "Beauty: How Will It Change Next?" *Vogue,* May, 1975.

———. "The Double Standard of Aging." *Saturday Review,* September, 1972.

———. "A Woman's Beauty: Put-Down or Power Source?" *Vogue,* April, 1975.

Stivers, Cyndi. "Jessica Lange: From Frog to Movie Princess." *Life,* March, 1983.

Stukane, Eileen. "After Mastectomy: How Women Cope." *Family Circle,* July 1, 1981.

Terkel, Studs. *American Dreams: Lost & Found.* New York: Pantheon Books, 1980.

The Undercover Story. New York: The Fashion Institute of Technology, 1982.
"The Unveiling of a New Ford." *Time,* October 23, 1978.
Vespa, Mary. "A Two-Year-Old in False Eyelashes." *Ms.,* September, 1976.
Wagatsuma, Erica, and Kleinke, Chris L. "Ratings of Facial Beauty by Asian-American and Caucasian Females." *Journal of Social Psychology,* December, 1979.
Walker, Alice. "When the Other Dancer Is the Self." *Ms.,* May, 1983.
Waters, Harry. "CBS's New Morning Star." *Time,* March 14, 1983.
"Weighing Traits of Prospective Mates." *Family Weekly,* March 26, 1983.
Weller, Sheila. "Ann-Margret—Fate Hasn't Been Kind but She's Still Fighting Back." *Ladies' Home Journal,* November, 1978.
"What's Wrong with a Bare Face?" *Glamour,* April, 1983.
Wheeler, Elizabeth. "The Perils of Pretty." *Working Woman,* May, 1981.
Wilson, Glenn, and Nias, David. "Beauty Can't Be Beat." *Psychology Today,* September, 1976.
Wiltshire, D. C. S. "Roman Aids to Beauty." *History Today,* May, 1979.
Wolkomir, Richard. "Personality Molds Your Looks—So Think Attractiveness." *Science Digest,* February, 1979.
"Women: What's on Their Minds? What's in Their Hearts? What Do They Fear? What Do They Hope For?" *Glamour,* January, 1983.
"Worry Scale: What We Fear Most and Least." *American Health,* September/October, 1983.
Yankelovich, Daniel. *New Rules: Searching for Self-Fulfillment in a World Turned Upside Down.* New York: Random House, 1981.

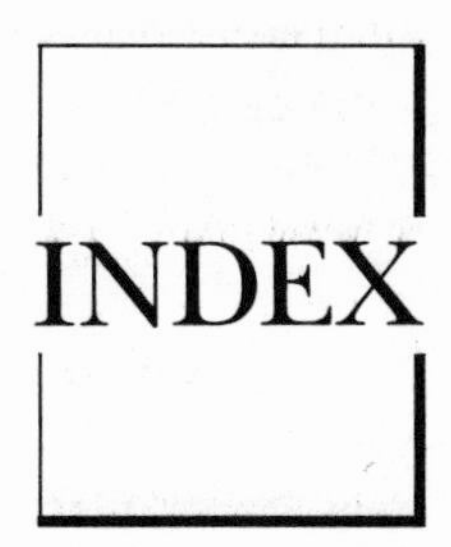

INDEX

CHICAGO HEIGHTS FREE PUBLIC LIBRARY
3 1539 00028 6179